A Study Guide

for

A More Excellent Way™

Pathways to Wholeness

HENRY W. WRIGHT

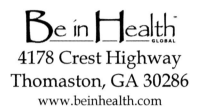

4178 Crest Highway
Thomaston, GA 30286
www.beinhealth.com

EAN 9-781934-680193 *A Study Guide* for *A More Excellent Way*™

Copyright Notice

Disclaimer

This ministry does not seek to be in conflict with any medical or psychiatric practices nor do we seek to be in conflict with any church and its religious doctrines, beliefs or practices. We are not a part of medicine or psychology, yet we work to make them more effective, rather than working against them. We believe many human problems are fundamentally spiritual with associated physiological and psychological manifestations. This information is intended for your general knowledge only. Information is presented only to give insight into disease, its problems and its possible solutions in the area of disease eradication and prevention. It is not a substitute for medical advice or treatment for specific medical conditions or disorders. You should seek prompt medical care for any specific health issues. Treatment modalities around your specific health issues are between you and your physician.*

As pastors, ministers and individuals of this ministry, we are not responsible for a person's disease, nor are we responsible for his or her healing. All we can do is share what we see about a problem. We are not professionals; we are not healers. We are only ministers ministering the Scriptures, and what they say about this subject, along with what the medical and scientific communities have also observed in line with this insight. There is no guarantee that any person will be healed or any disease be prevented. The fruit of this teaching will come forth out of the relationship between the person and God based on these insights, given and applied. This ministry is patterned after the following scriptures: 2 Corinthians 5:18-20; 1 Corinthians 12; Ephesians 4; Mark 16:15-20.

---

* Editor's Note: If you are taking prescription drugs, this ministry recommends that you do not come off of your medication without the supervision of a doctor.

Foreword

For centuries, healing has been a mystery to many Christians. But I believe heaven is closer to earth now than at any other time in history. As a result, we are obtaining clearer revelation about healing than ever before.

One example is *A More Excellent Way*™ by Pastor Henry W. Wright. His revelation of the spiritual roots of disease is revolutionary.

Several years ago, I interviewed a Jewish woman who had one of the worst cases of environmental illness I had ever heard about. As her condition deteriorated, she became allergic to plastic, clothing, and almost everything in the environment. Her allergic reactions were life threatening. When she visited Pastor Henry's ministry, she received a miraculous healing.

My friend, Kathryn Kuhlman, predicted that before Jesus returns, believers would be used by God to empty hospitals of the sick. Let's prepare by receiving all the revelation on healing that we can. For too long, Christians have been baffled and defeated by disease. There is *a more excellent way!*

Sid Roth, President
Messianic Vision, Inc.

Dedication

This Study Guide to accompany *A More Excellent Way*™, 7th Edition is dedicated to my mother, Norma Anne Wilson Wright, who went to be with the LORD, Thanksgiving Day, 1977. When I was in her womb, she was dying with fibrosarcoma cancer, fast growing and fatal. This cancer was wrapped around her jugular vein and had spread to large areas in her neck and up into the base of her brain. In this condition, paralyzed, wasting away and dying, she was present at a church service in Hatfield Point, New Brunswick, Canada, about two months after I was born. At this service God touched her, and she was instantly healed. Her doctors were unable to find any trace of the masses of cancer that they had observed previously. The cancer was gone! No medical treatment had been given. She lived for 34 more years, and was probably the only place of peace I ever had growing up. Her faith and her example and the testimony of her life continue to set an example for me, and not only for me, but for others who I will touch because of her steadfast faith in God. Her healing sets a standard within me against the enemy. Of a truth, God is no respecter of persons, and what He has done for one, He will do for another.

Appreciation

This appreciation is deeply expressed to Pastor Henry Wright for his work in researching God's Word and for God's divine gifts of love and mercy in revealing His healing message for His creation.

Pastor Henry has sought to be obedient every day since his calling, to establish a healing ministry and regain the lives lost to disease caused by the antichrist spirit. Scientists and the medical profession are now confirming his research in over 800 diseases.

His studies reveal the need for obedience to the Word of God by seekers of health and wholeness. His teachings and prayer models for healing are the result of this research and study. The healing message, ignored for hundreds of years in most churches since it was introduced by Jesus Christ, is again reaching people throughout the world.

Unnumbered volunteers, who have been healed and are now assisting this ministry throughout the world, join in this appreciation for Pastor Henry's work. The volunteers know who they are, as God also knows, whether here at Pleasant Valley Church or somewhere else, serving God and this ministry.

We give our appreciation and thanks to God for Pastor Henry Wright. Through his anointed message, we were healed by God. As a visionary, he is now changing the lives of those who need healing across the world.

He has also been honored to present messages across the United States, in Canada, in Africa and in the United Kingdom and Ireland, in Singapore, in Malaysia and in other countries. His messages and lectures have been recorded on television, radio, tape and DVD. His invitations to present this healing message are from all sizes and types of church groups, evangelical gatherings and special healing events.

Thank you, Pastor Henry Wright for helping change people's lives.

The Publishing Team
BE iN HEAlTh™

Preface

This Study Guide is designed to sow seeds of knowledge into your hearts about a big problem. The problem is spiritual, psychological and biological disease, and what we can do about it.

The format of the study guide follows the structure of *A More Excellent Way*™, 7th Edition and editions following. It includes page numbers from the book to assist the reader in locating answers to the study guide questions.

One of our desires is to better equip mankind with respect to defeating and preventing spiritual, psychological and biological disease. Also, one of our goals is to take away the mystery of disease and to be able to show from God's perspective why mankind has disease.

Over the years, God has shown us many insights into why mankind has disease. It is not that God cannot heal or that He does not want to. The problem is that man does not understand disease. We have gone into captivity and are perishing because of lack of knowledge, rejected knowledge or no knowledge at all. Investigation from science, the Scriptures, and our discernment has unearthed many spiritual roots and blocks to healing. In fact, the basic principles that, when applied, will move the hand of God to heal, are the same that, when applied, will prevent disease.

God's perfect will is not to heal you; His perfect will is that you do not get sick. Today, **Be iɴ Hᴇᴀʟᴛʜ**™ stands 100 percent for disease eradication and prevention, instead of disease management on a regular basis, if at all possible. To this end, **Be Iɴ Hᴇᴀʟᴛʜ**™ is dedicated.

This information should not be used as a method or a science or a formula or a quick fix to take the place of relationship with God. One of the main themes of this Study Guide is the connection between sin and disease. Another theme of the Study Guide is the consequences of separation from God, His Word, His love; separation from ourselves; and separation from others. One great concern for those using this book to try to help others is that they will make it into a science, or worse, use the knowledge in a legalistic manner to condemn others.

A heart of compassion is the key to ministry.

Table of Contents

Answers to unit questions are at the end of each unit.

Study Unit One:
My Purpose and Insight
See *A More Excellent Way*™, 7th Edition, pages 1 – 62˙

Introduction

When Pastor Henry began in ministry, he was part of a church that believed God was involved in people's lives, but even in that church, with the elders anointing them with oil, praying the prayer of faith, fasting and praying, and standing on the Word, people were not getting well from incurable diseases.

1. When Elders anoint with oil, pray in faith and fast with prayer and stand on the Word, does it always bring healing?   yes ___ no___

Jesus healed the people of their diseases and cast out their evil spirits. The disciples did it, the seventy did it, and the early church did it.

2. Is the church today in a dark age of time from which we have not recovered?   yes ___ no___

We do not see much sanctification of the body or soul or spirit. God's people struggle with the things of life as Paul did. Read Romans 7:14 to the end of the chapter. You will find Paul had major struggles with his own spirituality.

Paul said he had *sin* that dwelt *within* him. page 2

˙ Page numbers refer to *A More Excellent Way*™

3. Where does sin come from?

a. within us   b. outside of us

When Pastor Henry first became involved with people's lives, he prayed for them and believed God would heal them, but less than five percent of those he prayed for got well. God began to show His truth about disease from the Scriptures. It wasn't that He *could not* heal. It was that we had to become sanctified in certain areas of our lives before He *would* heal.

In the Old Testament, people were raised from the dead, people were healed, and many other miracles were done. In the New Testament, we have a new and better covenant. To be in health is better than receiving a healing.

> **Dearly beloved I wish above all things that you prosper and be in good health even as your soul prospers.**   3 John 1:2

It is God's will for us to *be in health*.

Sanctification is the process of becoming whole.

> **And the very God of peace sanctify you wholly; and I pray God your whole spirit and soul and body be preserved blameless unto the coming of our Lord Jesus Christ.**
> 1 Thessalonians 5:23

4. Being sanctified *wholly* affects what part of us?
   a. spirit   b. soul   c. body
   d. spirit, soul and body

Diseases in our lives can be the result of separation from God and His Word in specific areas of our lives. Except for those times when He would have mercy on whom He would have mercy, disease was an issue to do with circumcision of the heart.

> And he said, I will make all my goodness pass before thee, and I will proclaim the name of the LORD before thee; and will be gracious to whom I will be gracious, and will shew mercy on whom I will shew mercy. Exodus 33:19

> Therefore hath he mercy on whom he will have mercy, and whom he will he hardeneth. Romans 9:18

Many struggle with "gaps" between the Gospels (Matthew, Mark, Luke, John) and the other Epistles. After Acts, there is little discussion about healing and deliverance, causing some to say, "Well, it passed away because you do not find it." Or "Healing was only for Christ and the disciples but not for us."

In Matthew, Mark, Luke and John, the Lord demonstrated the love of God and power over the devil and disease in spite of sin. His disciples and the early church also demonstrated it in Acts. Then, from Romans all the way through Jude, you will find the Scriptures teaching us about *sanctification*.

The **Be in Health**™ Conferences taught across America and in other nations are really teaching sanctification in reverse. People do not attend conferences on holiness and sanctification as quickly as

3

they attend conferences on how the consequences of unrighteousness cause disease.

5. What is a New Testament scripture that mentions "cleansing the spirit?" _____

You cannot expect God to bless you if you are separated from Him in an area that needs to be dealt with. We have been taught much about God's promises, but not much about His Spirit of discernment and the consequences of sin.

6. Is discernment given to us by God?

yes_____ no_____
(Ask the Father for it!)

Eighty percent of incurable diseases have a spiritual root. A spiritual root is an internal, psychological or physiological effect of an unloving spirit.

7. Healing, to a degree, is conditional to your

_____. page 4

Does God forgive all manner of sin? Yes AND No. He wants to; that is His nature, but we can block Him.

**If we confess our sins, He is faithful and just
to forgive us our sins...** 1 John 1:9

After conversion,
there is an absolute requirement
and responsibility
to forgive others.
Is there anyone you need to forgive?

14For if ye forgive men their trespasses, your
heavenly Father will also forgive you:
15But if ye forgive not men their trespasses,
neither will your Father forgive your trespasses.
Matthew 6:14-15

So how do we resolve 1 John 1:9 with Matthew 6:14-15? page 5

Unforgiveness
may bind you to a disease.

8.   If we do not forgive others, what are the consequences? _____

9.   Just because you are born again and your spirit has become alive in God, it does not mean you have resolved the consequences of the _____ in your life.

God's perfect will is not to heal you.
God's perfect will is that you do not get sick.

The Lord's Prayer says,

Thy kingdom come. Thy will be done in
earth, as it is in heaven.   Matthew 6:10

In Deuteronomy 28 and Exodus 15, God promises that if we are obedient to Him none of the diseases of Egypt will fall upon us. page 7

5

10. Leviticus 13:9 instructed that if someone had leprosy, and later that person said he or she was clean, to whom were they sent to determine if they were healed? _____

11. James 5:14 says, if there be any sick among you, call whom? _____

*If you have been sick in the past,
what did you do first?
Pray or call the doctor?*

We think of sin as robbing banks, prostitution or lying and stealing. Would you consider **fear** to be sin? Would you consider **bitterness** to be sin? Would you consider **self-hatred** to be sin? Would you consider these things to be **sin**?

Fear is the number one plague of America, and it is the number one plague of the world —

fear of tomorrow	fear of disease
fear of death	fear of mothers-in-law
fear of man	fear of your neighbor
fear of dying	and on and on and on ...

Editor's Note: In the April 2, 2001 issue of *Time* Magazine, there is an article listing over 4,000 different types of fear.

*Our goal is disease prevention,
not disease management.*

12. How many of our diseases does God want to heal? _____ (Psalm 103:3)

Most of us know God is omnipotent, omniscient and omnipresent.

Many of us do not know Him as omnificent, all creative, ever able to fix that which needs to be fixed. Being omnificent makes Him magnificent — King of kings and Lord of all lords. He is God of all gods. He is the Creator of all flesh. He is the sustainer of all of mankind. page 10

It's not that God cannot heal you
or that He does not want to.
The problem is
that man does not understand disease.

We have gone into captivity and are perishing, either because of lack of knowledge or just no knowledge at all.

13. Who has "lack of knowledge?"

_____ (Isaiah 5:13) page 11

14. Who has "no knowledge?"

_____ (Hosea 4:6) page 11

Our "no knowledge" and "lack of knowledge" in the area of understanding is the relationship between sin and disease.

15. What is the greatest commandment?

_____

Scripture tells us to love the LORD thy God with all our heart.

> And thou shalt love the LORD thy God with all thine heart, and with all thy might.
> Deuteronomy 6:5
> But thou shalt love thy neighbor as thyself: I am the LORD.
> Leviticus 19:18

> [37]Jesus said unto him, Thou shalt love the Lord thy God with all thy heart, and with all thy soul, and with all thy mind.
> [38]This is the first and great commandment.
> [39]And the second is like unto it, Thou shalt love thy neighbour as thyself.
> Matthew 22:37-39

If you do not love yourself, you cannot love your neighbor. You may pretend you do.

Editor's Note: Your nearest neighbor is your spouse.

> *If married, pray about your relationship.*
> *Ask God if there is anything*
> *you need to change*
> *in your attitude*
> *or what you are doing.*

16. Is the husband supposed to be the spiritual leader and cover of the family? yes ___ no ___

Many people whose fathers are still alive are fatherless. Many women whose husbands are still alive are spiritual widows. page 13

FAITH vs. FEAR

Many people struggle with faith. Maybe you are sick, you have a disease, and you have been told you do not have enough faith. Maybe you have been listening to some of the people who teach that you need to do something to get more faith.

17. The Bible says in Romans 12:3 that every man (and woman) has been given a _____ of faith.

18. We need to be continually _____ by the washing of the water of the Word (2 Corinthians 4:16; Ephesians 5:26; 4:23; Colossians 3:10). pages 14-15

19. Romans 10:17 says faith comes by _____, and _____ by the Word of God.

20. Hebrews 11:1 says faith is the substance of things _____, the evidence of things not yet seen.

"Fear Faith" is not real faith. See *A More Excellent Way*™, 7th Edition, page 15. Faith projects into the future; fear also projects into the future.

21. Who is your enemy listed in Ephesians 6:11-12?
   _____

Autoimmune Disease

In the church, we sometimes attack each other. This is an autoimmune disease in the church!

> [34]A new commandment I give unto you, That ye love one another; as I have loved you, that ye also love one another.
> [35]By this shall all *men* know that ye are my disciples, if ye have love one to another.
>
> John 13:34-35

In Isaiah 58:1-4, the people of God were saying, "Hallelujah, LORD, we love you." **Yet they were destroying each other, and God would not protect them or hear them.**

That is the question of God's people in Isaiah 58. God said, "Yeah, I've watched you fasting and praying, **but you pray for strife, and eat each other alive. I have caused my ears to become deaf to you."** page 16

22. Why did God not heal them? _____

_____

God is saying (paraphrase): You want My blessings, but you do not want My friends. Do you realize that other person is a friend of Jesus? What do you think Jesus thinks about you talking that way about His friend? Do you think Jesus is our friend?

Jesus said,

> **Henceforth I call you not servants ... but I have called you friends.** John 15:15

Friends do not talk about each other. *Friends* build each other up. *Friends* cover with love. *Perfect love* covers a multitude of sins.

> **And above all things have fervent charity among yourselves: for charity shall cover the multitude of sins.** 1 Peter 4:8

23. Galatians 6:1 says that if a brother be overtaken in a fault, those of you who consider yourselves spiritual, _____such an one. Do not stone him by sundown. page 17

A sign of maturity is not just knowing what is good. It is knowing what is evil as well.

Hebrews 5:14 says, "Strong meat belongeth to them that are of full age, even those who by reason of use have their senses exercised to discern both good and evil."

We have been so God-conscious that we have forgotten *discernment concerning evil.* We have to know what is of God and what is not. That is a sign of maturity. page 18

24. Galatians 6:2 tells us to bear one another's _____ and so fulfill the law of Christ.

25. God says, Love your brother. Is restoring a brother part of loving him?   yes ___ no___

Recover yourself from the snare of the devil and be healed!

> [24]And the servant of the Lord must not strive; but be gentle unto all men, apt to teach, patient,
> [25]In meekness instructing those that oppose themselves; if God peradventure will give them repentance to the acknowledging of the truth;
> [26]And that they may recover themselves out of the snare of the devil, who are taken captive by him at his will.   2 Timothy 2:24-26

Discernment is required for freedom.
Promise without discernment is still bondage.

When people are in captivity by the devil, they do not know it. They do not understand. Why? No one has told them. The purpose of this ministry is to bring you insight and discernment that you may be recovered out of the snare of the devil.

Communion

In dealing with autoimmune disease, 1 Corinthians 11:29-31 is an example of a *block*, not a root, to healing:

> ²⁹For he that eateth and drinketh unworthily, eateth and drinketh damnation to himself, not discerning the Lord's body.
> ³⁰For this cause many are weak and sickly among you, and many sleep.
> ³¹For if we would judge ourselves, we should not be judged.   1 Corinthians 11:29-31

Many of God's people are weak and tired. Could that be like chronic fatigue syndrome?

26.   Does the word "sickly" mean "sick" to you?

yes ___ no ___

"Many sleep" does not mean they sleep in church; it means they die premature deaths.

Sometimes people are sick
because they do not rightly discern
the Lord's body.

If you are sick,
examine yourself concerning this teaching
to determine
if you are taking communion unworthily.

In Isaiah 58:1-4, God's people were destroying each other, and God refused to protect them or answer their prayers. page 21

27. Isaiah 58:4 says that we can fast for _____ and _____, and to smite with the fist of wickedness.

The fast of service in Isaiah 58 is not abstaining from food or water.

God called us to a fast
of service
to others in love.

The fast of service fulfills
all of Gods commandments to LOVE.

We do not have to be healed ourselves
in order to pray for another's healing.

28. Isaiah 58:6 says that God's chosen fast is to _____ the bands of wickedness, to undo the heavy _____, and to let the oppressed go _____ and to break every yoke.

Medication Insight

Many are ministering to the side effects of drugs, and wondering why God is not healing the problem. *USA Today* (April 24, 1998) contained an article about deadly drugs: "Why Are So Many Drugs Killing So Many Patients?"

29. "Adverse reactions to prescription drugs are the _____ largest cause of death nationally." page 24

Depression, Anxiety Attacks, and the Use of Prozac and Other Drugs

30. Many drugs are serotonin enhancers. A serotonin _____causes depression, migraines, binge eating, weight problems and obsessive-compulsive behavior (OCD). page 23

31. What is the root problem? _____ page 23

Somewhere, there has been a lack of nurturing in childhood. **Sometimes it can be inherited because the lack of nurturing has not been there from generation to generation.**

Prozac is the drug of choice today, yet it is sometimes prescribed without any thought of the consequences.

32. What are two side effects of Prozac? _____ and _____

For example, bipolar disorder may be associated with an *underproduction of serotonin* caused by a genetic

14

defect which produces a wide range of highs and lows from manic to depressive.

Migraines, binge eating, weight problems and obsessive-compulsive behavior (OCD) may also indicate an undersecretion of serotonin.

Would you be interested in a more excellent way?

This ministry is on the "cutting edge" of medicine in America.

33. Thousands of people are no longer on _____ _____ and are living normal lives because of their application of the teachings of the ministry. page 23

An article in *USA Today*, about deadly drugs lists the top ten killers in America:

#1 heart disease
#2 cancer
#3 strokes
#4 adverse drug reactions to prescription drugs
    (currently moved to number three)
#5 pulmonary disease
#6 accidents of all classes
#8 the medical profession

Death by *illegal* drugs does not even make this list, but death by *legally* prescribed drugs is on the top ten list!

Editor's Note:
    #7 pneumonia and influenza (currently replaced by diabetes)
    #9 HIV and AIDS
    #10 suicide

There is *a more excellent way* through the gifts of the Spirit and faith in God.

34. The children of Israel did not enter the promised land because they did not mix _____ with the gospel they had received. (Hebrews 3:19-4:2) page 25

That is the first reason; the second reason is they did not enter into their rest (as God entered into His rest in creation on the seventh day). They did not cease from their own labors.

35. Is drivenness a fruit of the Spirit?

yes ___ no ___

The devil *drives* and God *leads*. page 25

> **For as many as are *led* by the Spirit of God,**
> **they are the sons of God.**   Romans 8:14

Understand how God thinks.
Apply how God thinks
to your own thoughts and actions.

Pastor Henry has concluded that 80 percent of *all* diseases in America and in the world, which have the name *syndrome* or *incurable* attached to it, have a spiritual root.

We cannot
bypass the penalty of sin
in our lives.

This ministry advocates a good balanced diet. However, good nutrition, rest and drinking enough water by themselves do not heal the defects that come because of separation from God and His Word, or deal with sanctification, sin and the resulting diseases. pages 302 – 303

36. Nutrition does not replace _____.

37. How many of our diseases does He heal in Psalm 103? _____

Jesus tied the lack of sanctification to disease when He said in John 14, "Sin no more lest a worse thing come unto thee." God wants to heal us.

> **Who forgiveth all thine iniquities; who healeth all thy diseases;** Psalm 103:3

Notice that iniquity comes before disease in this scripture.

> **Beloved, I wish above all things that thou mayest prosper and be in health, even as thy soul prospereth.** 3 John 1:2

Editor's note: Be In Health™, the official name of the ministry of Pastor Henry W. Wright, was taken from this scripture.

> **And the very God of peace sanctify you wholly; and *I pray God* your whole spirit and soul and body be preserved blameless unto the coming of our Lord Jesus Christ.**
> 1 Thessalonians 5:23

We have become separated from God in our understanding of disease. Refer above to "Who does the scripture say to take the sick to?" in this Unit. page 27

> **14Is any sick among you? let him call for the elders of the church; and let them pray over him, anointing him with oil in the name of the Lord:**

17

> ¹⁵**And the prayer of faith shall save the sick, and the Lord shall raise him up; and if he have committed sins, they shall be forgiven him.**
>
> James 5:14-15

In these verses we see the lack of sanctification in a believer's life and the consequence. This shows us the relationship of sin to disease.

Many times the church quotes James 5:14 and drops off James 5:15 which says "...if he have committed sins." When God does not heal, it is because He cannot do so without giving us a leavened gospel that would say we could keep our sin and receive His blessings.

The Doctrine of Balaam

Pastor Henry believes that the doctrine of Balaam is in the church today. The doctrine of Balaam teaches there are no consequences for sin.

Read Numbers 22-24, 31; 2 Peter 2:15; Jude 11; Revelation 2:14. What came? **The curse came.** There was no longer any provision for safety, and 24,000 Israelites died in the plague that came as the result of their sin. page 28

38. The church has come to a place where they have overplayed grace and mercy to the point that they say, "Because you are in covenant, you can sin like the devil, and there are no consequences." This ministry disagrees. We have to get _____ and remain under the conviction of the Holy Spirit every single day to become more holy. page 29

Some teach, "You never have to repent again once you are saved." This ministry disagrees!

If you sin against your brother, then go and repent to your brother.

Matthew 18:15 says that if you have ought (anger) against your brother, you go to your brother alone. (Also see Matthew 5:22-24.) page 29

The following scripture is addressed to the saints, not to the heathen.

> ...dearly beloved, let us cleanse ourselves from all filthiness of the flesh and spirit.
>
> 2 Corinthians 7:1

As you are in covenant with God,
the principles you apply to your life
that will move His hand to heal you
are the same principles that,
if you apply them to your life,
will prevent disease in your life.

Wrong Doctrine

Some teach, "Disease is from God." If that is true, then Jesus was out of God's will when He healed in Acts 10:38.

> How God anointed Jesus of Nazareth with the Holy Ghost and with power: who went about doing good, and healing all that were oppressed of the devil; for God was with him.
>
> Acts 10:38

If you meet people who say their disease is from God, ask them if they are going to a doctor. When they tell you, "Yes," say to them, "If you really believe God gave you this disease, why are you trying to get rid of it by going to a doctor?"

Recognize your spiritual issues (roots).
Remove any blocks to healing
by recognizing them,
taking responsibility, repenting
and asking God to forgive you.

The Spirit of Fear

Second Timothy 1:7 tells us that God has not given us a spirit of fear, but He has given us power, love and a sound mind.

All three members of the Godhead are present in this scripture:

- **Power — Who is the power of God? God, the Holy Spirit.**

- **Love — Who is the love factor? God, the Father.**

- **Sound Mind — Who is the sound mind? God, Jesus, The Son.**

What is the antidote to fear? A relationship with the whole Godhead: fellowship with the Father, fellowship with Jesus, who is the Word, and fellowship with the Holy Spirit as He indwells you. You then will not have any fear. You will be hanging out with God.

Do you think that is *a more excellent way?*

When we minister to people and they are not healed, what do you think we ought to do? Make up a theology that God does not heal today or that someone did not have enough faith? Do we go into unbelief and doubt? There is a spiritual root or a block to healing that has to be dealt with.

See "Blocks to Healing" in *A More Excellent Way*™, 7th Edition, page 253.

When we minister to people and they are not healed, we should do what Pastor Henry does. Go back to God and say, "Why not? You better talk to me, Boss. Why weren't they healed?" Many times there is a reason that healing did not happen. See 2 Timothy 2:24-26. page 32

Fear is Sin

When we deal with allergies, simple and multiple, we tell people, "When the spies came into the promised land, what was the land filled with? Dairy products, sugar and wheat." (Numbers 13:27)

39. First Timothy 4:4-5 tells us our food is
_____ by the Word of God and prayer.

*At every meal, with thanksgiving,
ask God to bless and sanctify your food.*

Every meal pray over your food and give thanks.

Restore

Restore those who are in prison houses and are a prey to the beast of the field. Deliver them. Restore them.

40. Scripture says in 2 Chronicles 16:9 that the eyes of the Lord run to and fro throughout the whole earth, to show Himself _____ in behalf of them whose heart is perfect toward Him.

The Lord has not changed, but the church has.

In Jeremiah 2:8 we read,

> **The priests said not, Where *is* the LORD...**
> Jeremiah 2:8

Look at Jeremiah 6:13-14 concerning the spiritual condition of the Old Testament church and its leadership. page 35

Later on in chapter 8, Jeremiah again picks up the theme that says the same thing all over again.

Jeremiah 3:14 says,

> **Turn, oh backsliding children, saith the LORD...** Jeremiah 3:14

Some things to consider:

- Are we rightly discerning the Lord's body in communion?

- Are we repenting and being delivered from the snare of the devil?

- Are we forgiving those who hurt us?

Spiritual Husband

The Lord is your spiritual husband. You guys have a husband, not in the carnal, human standpoint, but in the mystical standpoint of His being our Master forever. (See Revelation 19:7; 22:17.)

41. We are all called the _____ of Christ. page 36

> They have healed also the hurt *of the daughter* of my people slightly, saying, Peace, peace; when *there is* no peace. Jeremiah 6:14

Today there are many sermons about God being our peace, but there are as many believers on Prozac as there are unbelievers on Prozac. Prozac is a cheap substitute for the Holy Spirit, who is called the Comforter by the Lord.

We are not going to say peace, peace when there isn't any. We are going to come before God, find where the bondage is, where the roots are, where the blocks are and get right before God, so that the Scriptures can be fulfilled.

Jesus said,

> Peace I leave with you, my peace I give unto you: not as the world giveth, give I unto you. Let not your heart be troubled, neither let it be afraid. John 14:27

Why Are Some Not Healed?

Sometimes you can have two people with the same sin and the same identical disease, and one is healed and the other is not. Why?

The difference is often in their attitude toward sin.

42. Your _____ toward God concerning sin is what moves Him. page 38

If you have a hatred for sin, even if you are still in your sin, God judges you according to the righteousness of your heart toward Him.

Some people, when confronted with sin, harden their hearts, and are not convicted; they do not have a perfect hatred for it.

God is going to judge the intent of your heart.

In Romans 7:15-17, we saw that the Apostle Paul also struggled with the issue of sin in his life.

Refer to the *7 Steps to Sin* (James 1:12-16) in Appendix B, *A More Excellent Way*™, 7th Edition.

Temptation is not sin.

Many people, because they are *tempted*, feel that they have sinned. You only have sin when the action of that sin is fulfilled; then it becomes your sin.

Many say, "Well, I'll just go ahead and do it because I've already thought about it." This is Satan's snare to convince you that the temptation equals the act.

How do we correct a wrong when the person is dead?

Many people are bound by disease because of unresolved issues concerning people who have died.

God judges the matter by your heart. If you have something from your past and it is not possible for you to make it right with the person, then you make it right with God and it is taken care of. You do not have to carry the guilt any longer.

If people are holding a sin against you, it is *their* problem, not yours. They have to get it right before God just like you do. Whether they do or they don't really does not have anything to do with you, because you are standing *alone* before God in the integrity of *your* heart.

If you have a breach with someone,
and the person will not talk to you or make peace with you,
your ability to be free of that situation
does not mean you have to resolve it personally
with that person.

You can come before God.
He will work with your heart,
but you do not have to have it resolved
with anyone in order to be free.

You have to have it resolved before God.
Your heart has to make the paradigm shift
concerning this issue.

Conflict Resolution

If you have been victimized…

You do not have to resolve one issue with someone that has victimized you in order for God to heal you, providing you have resolved that issue between you and God concerning the person.

43. If you are waiting for resolution between you and the other person before you can be well, you have bought a _____. page 40

All of us shall stand before God one day, and we cannot say, "They made me do it. They made me do it." **You will stand alone before God.**

Victimization

How do you honor your parents, or husband, or wife, (or children,) when they constantly "beat you up" in some manner? There are many people condemned by the scripture that says to honor your mother and your father (Matthew 19:19)...

You only have to honor mother or father or anyone to the degree that they honor God!

Now, you cannot touch [dishonor] them either, but you do not have to go along with their sin.

Some people tell me: "I just do not want to talk about what my mother did to me or my father did to me because that is not honoring them."

No, that is not about honoring them — it is just defining the evil. You do not have to honor the evil in parents. We cannot afford to preach a gospel that produces a codependency with evil.

Codependency
is calling evil good in the name of love.

However, the first thing that you must be able to do is separate them from their sin.

Psalm 97:10 says,

> **Ye that love the LORD, hate evil: he preserveth the souls of his saints; he delivereth them out of the hand of the wicked.**
>
> Psalm 97:10

If you are around a good body of believers where there are some good fathers and mothers in the Lord, I pray that God gives them to you quickly. They can fill you up with the love you need. Women, you can begin to realize Jesus is your husband to be.

In a victimization situation, whether it is children, or husbands, or wives, this ministry recommends immediate separation and never sends a wife back to an abusive husband.

Give those who have wronged you to the Lord; you do not have to fix them.

*In the past,
when people behaved
in an evil manner against us,
we believed them to be evil.*

*After this teaching, when people are evil to you,
separate them from their sin.*

See Unit Four on Separation.

Separation from abusive situations is godly, not ungodly. There may be a time, after you have been sanctified and strengthened in the area of your weaknesses that you can go back into the situation and be all right.

When Pastor Henry ministers to children who have been subjected to victimization, he says that the worst thing he can do is send them back to the abusive parent. His position is that all victims are removed immediately until the one victimizing decides *where his (or her) treasure is.*

44. If you go back into a *victimization* situation in the name of love, it is called _____. page 44

Ten Commandments of Successful Relationships

1. Communicate	6. Communicate
2. Communicate	7. Communicate
3. Communicate	8. Communicate
4. Communicate	9. Communicate
5. Repent	10. Repent

45. The root problem of misunderstandings is that someone did not _____ .

**With freedom
comes great responsibility.**

46. First Corinthians 13:12 says,
For now we see through a glass _____ .

So, we are turning on a light in that darkness. With a better life comes responsibility and conditions. Freedom requires an effort.

> **Submit yourselves therefore to God. Resist the devil, and he will flee from you.** James 4:7

Resisting requires an effort. It is God that does the work in us, but we have to participate.

> **For I have no pleasure in the death of him that dieth, saith the Lord GOD: wherefore *turn yourselves*, and live ye.** Ezekiel 18:32

> **Having therefore these promises, dearly beloved, let us cleanse ourselves from all filthiness of the flesh and spirit, perfecting holiness in the fear of God.** 2 Corinthians 7:1

*In each of these verses,
an action is required on our part.*

Have you ever heard that voice in your head that tells you how rotten you are, and that you are a failure, and always will be?

**Condemnation is of the devil.
Conviction is because of God's love for us.**

From glory to glory, we are being changed into His image.

> But we all, with open face beholding as in a glass the glory of the Lord, are changed into the same image from glory to glory, *even* as by the Spirit of the Lord.   2 Corinthians 3:18

The work of God in the earth today is one of sanctification. Often you will not receive healing and deliverance from God without first submitting to God.

> Humble yourselves therefore under the mighty hand of God, that he may exalt you in due time.   1 Peter 5:6

> Seek ye first the kingdom of God and His righteousness and all these things shall be added unto you.   Matthew 6:33

47. Matthew, Mark, Luke, John and the book of Acts are a demonstration of God's love through the Lord and through the apostles in the early church. From Romans to Jude, God deals with our s_____tif_____n.

Jungian Psychology

Hebrews 4:12 teaches us that the soul and the spirit are distinctively separate.

> For the word of God *is* quick, and powerful, and sharper than any twoedged sword, piercing even to the dividing asunder of soul and spirit, and of the joints and marrow, and *is* a discerner of the thoughts and intents of the heart.
> Hebrews 4:12

It says, "Is able to separate the spirit from the soul." One of the great tragedies of psychology in the teaching of Jungian psychology is that it eliminates the *spirit of man* totally and inserts in its place the dualistic compartments of the soul.

In Jungian psychology and in modern day psychology, there is no such thing as the spirit of man.

There are the dualistic compartments of the soul called the "conscious" and the "collective unconscious." In the teachings of Jungian psychology, within the collective unconscious, you will find the archetypes and dark shadows. Jungian psychology identifies these dark shadows as the archetypes of our historic ancestry, bringing with them the darkness and the evil that we need to come in contact with, and identify with, so that we can cohabit with the evil of our ancestral line, generationally. This is classic Jungian psychotherapy.

I do not find these concepts anywhere in Scripture. What I do find in Scripture is that the archetypes and dark shadows are, in fact, evil spirits, principalities, powers and the rulers of the darkness of this world.

> **For we wrestle not against flesh and blood, but against principalities, against powers, against the rulers of the darkness of this world, against spiritual wickedness in high *places*.**
> Ephesians 6:12

48. Carl Jung became a channeler for invisible entities. In his writings, the principal entity that he channeled was a spirit entity called
_____.

He also channeled two lesser spirit entities called Anima and Animus, who became the foundation of the male and female principles in Jungian psychology. This male-female principle can even be found in Christian ministry and counseling circles as a therapeutic model.

This means that much of modern Jungian psychology was written by invisible spirit beings. In his early writings, Carl Jung called them evil spirits. As he developed his precepts, he said, "Because of the failure of Christianity in dealing with the problems of the psyche or the soul of man, and the body, or the diseases of man, *I will create an alternative to Christianity*," because He considered Christianity to be a dead religion. Modern-day psychology includes many Jungian principles and is the fruit of the failure of the Christian church.

We are not into inner healing as it is taught by certain practitioners. I go far beyond that. We are into the sanctification of the human spirit.

We are familiar with Hebrews 4:12, but most people overlook Hebrews 4:13.

> **Neither is there any creature that is not manifest in his sight: but all things *are* naked and opened unto the eyes of him with whom we have to do.** Hebrews 4:13

Satan's domain is the second heaven.

The manifested creatures, and naked things, are Satan's kingdom of the second heaven that are trying to rule mankind. They are the principalities and powers, spiritual wickedness in high places and the rulers of darkness of Ephesians 6:12. They are the archetypes and dark shadows of Jungian psychology. The church is incredibly ignorant about its enemy.

Paul said,

I was caught up to the third heaven.
2 Corinthians 12:2

If there is a first heaven and a third heaven, what comes in between? The second heaven. Satan is called the prince of the power of the air.

Wherein in time past ye walked according to the course of this world, according to the prince of the power of the air, the spirit that now worketh in the children of disobedience:
Ephesians 2:2

Teaching on Memory

We think on two levels. Your spirit man thinks and your intellect thinks independently of your spirit man.

Hebrews 4:12 tells us the Word of God comes to separate the soul from the spirit. Why? **To get God's Word to enter into your human spirit so your mind is renewed by the washing of the water of the Word.**

49. As a work of the Holy Spirit who shall lead you into all truth, your spirit and your soul now _____ _____ in God's way of thinking and following God.

In the process of becoming one in God's way of thinking, there is a gap that has to be worked out. This is the stuff that does not want to let you change your way of thinking. Changing your thinking is really scary because your mind will pitch a fit.

50. How is your soul saved? Your brain cells are part of your soul. When you die, your brain cells die with your body, but the _____ _____ of the _____ thoughts remain with your spirit which returns to God to await the resurrection.

This is how it works. We have both short-term and long-term memory which are made up of units of memory called "memes." You have individual memes, you have mass memes, and you have thoughts remaining with your spirit, which returns to God to await the resurrection.

51. When people have a broken heart and their spirit has been injured, **we minister to remove the pain in the heart.** After the Lord comes to heal, they have the _____ in the mind, but the _____ in the heart no longer exists. How is that?

What was removed was the creature inside, spiritually, that was reinforcing the damage and the thought. (Hebrews 12:13)

Behind spiritually rooted diseases are always feelings, emotions and thoughts. Your enemy is banking on the fact that he has captured your mind. He has to have you, because without you his kingdom cannot exist on this planet. (Genesis 3)

**The enemy wants to use you
as a medium of expression.
People are channelers for the devil
and do not even know it.**

52. When you hate your brother, you are a
_____ for the devil. When you slander
your brother, you are an oracle for Satan.

This is why your mind needs to be renewed by
the washing of the water of the Word.

> And be renewed in the spirit of your mind...
> Ephesians 4:23
> That he might sanctify and cleanse it with the
> washing of water by the word. Ephesians 5:26

In short-term memory you "take a picture" — that
is a meme, but it does not become fixed. A unit of
memory is an electrical, chemical occurrence that
happens in the brain. In long-term memory we have
something that happens that is now being *reinforced*: by
meditation, by *repetition* and by a *locking in of
consciousness*, so that something happens in the
electrochemical occurrence.

53. There is a factor of genetics that occurs involving
RNA. Something called protein synthesis occurs,
and that memory becomes _____ a
part of your brain cells, not just as a flash point or
a picture in short-term memory.

That is how your soul is preserved. The mirror
image is taken like a negative. The human spirit picks it
up, and you become one with it spiritually and
psychologically.

My will should match the Father's will, and my word should match the Word of God, and my actions should be as if they were the Holy Spirit. So the will and the Word and the action of God can be performed through me as a way of life. I am to be a total extension of the Word, the will and the action. Isn't it amazing that we have been created in God's image?

Some of you have been *conforming* to the mind of Satan, the mind of death, the mind of antichrist and to things that are diametrically *opposed to what God says.*

We usually do things by just thinking about them first.

The three members of the eternal Godhead are in perfect agreement. The Father wills it. The Word says it, and the Holy Spirit does it.

If you are in fellowship with the Godhead and if you are in fellowship with God by His Word, you should be: *an extension of the will, the Word and the power of God as a way of life.*

When the world sees you, they ought to see an extension of the Godhead at every point they turn. Would that be something idealistic to think about or do you think that is scriptural? He wants you well, in your right mind, in health, sanity and to be the fulfillment of 1 Thessalonians 5:23.

> And the very God of peace sanctify you wholly; and I pray God your whole spirit and soul and body be preserved blameless unto the coming of our Lord Jesus Christ.
>
> 1 Thessalonians 5:23

Sanctification means the burning fire of the Holy Spirit, which brings conviction and makes you whole.

God wants to sanctify you wholly in spirit, soul and body.

God does not just want you fixed in one dimension; He wants you fixed in every dimension of your creation. **It begins deep on the inside.**

As he thinketh in his heart, so *is* he...
Proverbs 23:7

Biblical Standard for Healing

We have established, first of all, the biblical standard for healing. It is God's will to get involved in your life.

The second thing we established is that the church has been a miserable failure in dealing with it.

Number three, from the prophet in Ezekiel 34, we established that God the Father, by the Spirit of God, revealed that He was ticked off about it, and He had a few things to say against the spiritual leaders: They were not healing the sick; they were not taking care of the diseased; and they were not searching for the ones who were lost over the cliff.

We also found, in both the Old Testament and the New Testament, that it is God's will for us to prosper in spirit, soul and body.

This ministry deals with the etiology of over 600 different, so-called incurable diseases in America and the world.

Saying the word "incurable" makes the devil greater than God.

We believe all things are possible. Mankind has disease because we have become separated from God and His Word and fallen into disobedience to Him. All disease that has a spiritual root is a result of the lack of sanctification in our lives as men and women of God, and all healing and prevention of disease is the process of being re-sanctified.

Remember Thessalonians says,

> **May the God of peace sanctify you wholly in spirit, in soul and in body.**   1 Thessalonians 5:23

God is not going to bless us and let us keep our sin. This is not legalism. This is not about the *works* of righteousness. This is a *heart* change — the circumcision of the human heart, the submission to the living God because we want to submit, not because we have to.

There is a connection between sin and disease as it says in Deuteronomy 28. Disobedience to God and His Word and not staying in covenant with Him will open the door to the curse. In Deuteronomy 28, in the section on curses, we find all manner of disease. But when men came into obedience to God and His Word, and in covenant with Him and His children, we found blessings. There was not one disease listed.

This ministry considers all disease to be a curse and not a blessing. This ministry considers all absence of disease to be a blessing.

Deuteronomy 30:19-20 tells us to choose this day what we shall have, blessings or curses, life or death. page 58

Psalm 103:3 addresses forgiveness of sin and healing of disease.

54. Psalm 103:3 says "Who forgiveth _____ thine iniquities; who healeth _____ thy diseases.

In one verse, we have both forgiveness of sin and healing of disease together.

> [14]Is any sick among you? Let him call for the elders of the church: and let them pray over him, anointing him with oil in the name of the Lord: [15]And the prayer of faith shall save the sick, and the Lord shall raise him up; and if he have committed sins, they shall be forgiven him.
> James 5:14-15

> Afterward Jesus findeth him in the temple, and said unto him, Behold, thou art made whole: sin no more, lest a worse thing come unto thee.
> John 5:14

Lack of Sanctification and Disease

Right here in the harmony of just three scriptures, I see a direct relationship between lack of sanctification, disease and sin.

In 2 Chronicles 29 and 30, the people had been serving pagan gods, and Hezekiah came as the Levite priests offered sacrifices for sin. Worship went up to God. The LORD heard and He healed, but sanctification had to occur first.

> And the LORD hearkened to Hezekiah, and
> healed the people.   2 Chronicles 30:20

In order for you to be able to come to a place of receiving healing from God, you have to be in fellowship with all three members of the Godhead: the Father, the Lord (Jesus the Son) and the Holy Spirit.

> The grace of the Lord Jesus Christ, and the
> love of God, and the communion of the Holy
> Ghost, be with you all. Amen.   2 Corinthians 13:14

55. Much of the church body today is trying to receive from God through prayers and petitions, but they are not in fellowship; they are not in _____. Jesus said loving Him requires obeying Him.

> If ye love me, keep my commandments.
> John 14:15

Out of the fellowship comes worship. We worship the Father and the Son, who is Jesus. The work of the Holy Spirit is to confirm and execute the will of the Father and the Word of God.

> [13]Howbeit when he, the Spirit of truth, is come, he will guide you into all truth: for he shall not speak of himself; but whatsoever he shall hear, that shall he speak: and he will shew you things to come.
> [14]He shall glorify me: for he shall receive of mine, and shall shew it unto you.
> [15]All things that the Father hath are mine: therefore said I, that he shall take of mine, and shall shew it unto you.   John 16:13-15

56. All good things come down _____ the _____, in the _____ of Jesus, as a work of the Holy Spirit.

> Every good gift and every perfect gift is from above, and cometh down from the Father of lights, with whom is no variableness, neither shadow of turning.   James 1:17

57. That is why we go to the Father, in the name of Jesus, and the Holy Spirit performs it. We are only to contact _____ member of the Godhead in petition.

> 23And in that day ye shall ask me nothing. Verily, verily, I say unto you, Whatsoever ye shall ask the Father in my name, he will give *it* you.
> 24Hitherto have ye asked nothing in my name: ask, and ye shall receive, that your joy may be full.   John 16:23-24

Pastor Henry said, "I do not see a well church trying to save a sick world. I see a sick church trying to save itself. It should be a well church trying to save a sick world."

Reestablish your relationship with God, and you will be in worship. When fellowship and worship are in place, and you come before God, in the name of the Lord, you will have His attention. It will cost you nothing.

Maybe you will be one of the people who hear this and are never the same because when you applied these principles, and went before God and the Word, you walked away from certain diseases just like you never had them. You have to work out your problems, do that circumcision, do that repentance, get before God, get back into fellowship, and get to a place where you are going to be honest with God about your problem, and deal with it.

The Bible says,

> If the Son therefore shall make you free, ye
> shall be free indeed.   John 8:36

Knowing God's Word

When we get into certain difficulties, we find that at some point in our family trees or in our own lives, our minds and our spirits have been opened up to the other kingdom. We have listened to those voices, and we have followed modalities of thought and precepts that are diametrically opposed to what God has said in His Word.

**The biggest problem that I find
in the Christian church today
is that Christians
do not know the Word of God.**

> Study to shew thyself approved unto God, a
> workman that needeth not be ashamed, rightly
> dividing the word of truth.   2 Timothy 2:15

That is where you begin. Then take God's Word and mix it with your faith, and take it into your heart. You will never be the same, and you will change your life, your family's lives, your city, your church and your world.

The revealed will of God and the living Word for mankind to follow can be found in the pages of

Scripture. When we follow other ways of thinking, or other gods or other spiritual leaders, we have opened up our spirits to forces that are designed to steal our faith and bring us torment.

**All fear comes
from not trusting God
and His Word.**

Be careful for nothing; but in everything by prayer and supplication with thanksgiving let your requests be made known unto God.
Philippians 4:6

If our minds, spirits and souls are filled with fear and confusion, projection and avoidance, we are no earthly good today. Forget the past and forget the future.

*Let God be God
in your life today!*

Take therefore no thought for the morrow: for the morrow shall take thought for the things of itself. Sufficient unto the day is the evil thereof. Matthew 6:3

Answers to Unit One

1. no

2. yes

3. a. from within

4. d. spirit, soul and body

5. 2 Corinthians 7:1

6. yes

7. obedience

8. disease

9. sin issues

10. the priests

11. the elders

12. all

13. God's people

14. God's people

15. love the Lord thy God, love thyself, love others

16. yes

17. measure

18. renewed

19. hearing, hearing

20. hoped for

21. principalities, powers, rulers of darkness of this world, spiritual wickedness in high places

22. they were fasting for strife

23. restore

24. burdens

25. yes

26. yes

27. strife, debate

28. loose, burdens, free

29. fourth

30. deficiency

31. lack of self-esteem, self-rejection, self-hatred, guilt

32. anxiety and loss of libido

33. prescription drugs

34. faith

35. no

36. repentance

37. all

38. sanctified

39. sanctified

40. strong

41. bride

42. attitude

43. lie

44. codependency

45. understand

46. darkly

47. sanctification

48. Philemon

49. become one

50. mirror image, soul

51. memory, pain

52. oracle

53. biologically

54. all, all

55. obedience

56. from, Father, name

57. one

Study Unit Two:
Spiritually Rooted Disease

See *A More Excellent Way*™, 7th Edition, pages 63-93*

Mankind has disease, first of all, because we are separated from God, His Word, His truth and His love. Does that include members of His church? Yes. There seems to be no difference between the church and the world.

The purpose of this teaching is to bring you to a place of focus so that you may recover yourself from the snare of the devil, not only for the healing of disease, but for the prevention of it.

Spiritually rooted disease is the result of separation from God, His Word and His Love.

The character of God the Father may not have been shown to you by your earthly father. The true character of God the Father is also different from the "religious" God we have heard about that finds fault with our behavior and punishes us.

How can we know the Father's true character? We can know His true character from His Word.

The Old Testament tells us that God the Father is the head of the government of God. The position of the Father is one of authority over the Godhead. It is not

---

* Page numbers refer to *A More Excellent Way*™

within God's character to abuse or neglect us. Even in His position of authority, He always remains true to His character.

The order of the Godhead and His government in the third heaven is:

1. First, God the _____.

2. Second, God the _____ that came in the flesh as Jesus.

3. Third, God the _____ _____.

The Book of Psalms says,

> **Blessed be the Lord, who daily loadeth us with benefits, even the God of our salvation. Selah.** Psalm 68:19

4. John 14:9b says,
   > He that hath seen me hath seen _____.

5. John 5:30 says,
   > I can of mine own self do nothing: as I hear, I judge: and my judgment is just; because I seek not mine own will, but the will of the _____ which hath sent me.

6. John 5:19 says,
   > The Son can do nothing of himself, but what he seeth the _____ do: for what things soever he doeth, these also doeth the Son likewise.

7. James 1:17 says,
   > Every good gift and every perfect gift is from above, and cometh down from the _____ of lights, with whom is no variableness, neither shadow of turning.

8.   The Lord's prayer in Matthew 6:9 says,
     Our _____ who art in heaven...

9.   Jesus said in John 16:23,
     ...in that day you will ask me nothing.
     Verily, verily I say to you, Whatsoever you shall
     ask the _____in My name, he will
     give it you.

10. Jesus said in John 10:30,
     My_____ and I are One.

If your earthly father
abused his position of authority over you,
would you be willing
to let someone stand in his place
to minister the Father's Love to you?

Use the following model
for Ministry of the Father's Love.

Ministry Model for the Father's Love

How to Minister Healing
to Those Who Were Not Loved by Their Fathers

1. To minister healing, you need a man who is willing to represent God the Father and show His love to this person. Be sensitive to the Holy Spirit.

2. Introduce yourself to the person receiving ministry.

3. Greet the person using his or her name. Look for a name tag.

4. Then say:

    *   I, as your Christian brother, am going to take responsibility this day for a father who would not or could not say, "I love you."

    *   Will you forgive your father for not telling you that he loved you? (Matthew 6:24)

    *   Can you come to the place where you forgive your father for those things he did or didn't do? Release your father to God to deal with his issues. Release him and forgive him.

    *   In the name of Jesus Christ of Nazareth, I release you from that pain. We ask the Holy Spirit to come and heal your broken heart, and when He does, fear that entered when your heart was broken, has to go. (1 John 4:18)

- This day you will hear these words in your heart:

  "I love you."

  "I am glad you were born."

  "I am proud of you."

  "You are a good son (or daughter)."

5. When you are finished, hold the person. Do not talk. Just hold him or her until God has healed their broken heart.

> He healeth the broken in heart, and bindeth up their wounds.   Psalms 147:3
>
> The Spirit of the Lord is upon me, because he hath anointed me to preach the gospel to the poor; he hath sent me to heal the brokenhearted, to preach deliverance to the captives, and recovering of sight to the blind, to set at liberty them that are bruised,   Luke 4:18
>
> The Spirit of the Lord GOD is upon me; because the LORD hath anointed me to preach good tidings unto the meek; he hath sent me to bind up the brokenhearted, to proclaim liberty to the captives, and the opening of the prison to them that are bound;   Isaiah 61:1

Separation from Yourself

11. Separation from self happens when you struggle with self-hatred, lack of self-esteem and _____. How can you not love yourself if God loves you?

**All autoimmune diseases are the result
of refusing to believe
what God has said about your value.**

Lupus, Crohn's, diabetes, rheumatoid arthritis and MS are a few examples of autoimmune diseases coming out of *separation from self.*

12. All _____ diseases have a spiritual root of self-hatred, self-bitterness and guilt.

When we do not love ourselves:

- We oppose *God.*

- We listen to and believe another gospel.

- We make ourselves a "god unto ourselves."

- We deny His statement of love. What has God said in His Word and by His Spirit about our value?

- We open the door and invite the enemy and his kingdom to join with us in our spirit.

A human lifespan, according to God's prophesy through Moses (Psalm 90:10-12), is 70-80 years. Anything less than that is the result of a curse. Moses' ministry began at age 80!

If God loves you, what gives you the authority to say He is wrong? He is greater than you are. He who is greatest and holiest of all, God the Father, says He loves you.

Which gospel are you listening to?
If thoughts come to your mind telling you
how stupid, or worthless, or guilty you are,
these thoughts are coming from your enemy.

If you believe a disease is incurable,
are you believing the truth
about God and His sovereignty?

If you have accepted
self-hatred, self-bitterness and guilt,
then turn to Appendix C
and follow the Ministry Prayer Model.

Separation from Others

When you have bitterness (unforgiveness) toward others, that bitterness separates you from them and causes fragmentation in your spirit and in your soul. It is also the spiritual root behind many physical diseases.

Forgiving others allows us to heal.
Forgiveness is necessary for disease prevention.

What are we actually doing when we forgive ourselves and others? When we forgive ourselves and others, we are making a choice to participate with God to prevent disease.

Think of someone who has wronged you.
Do you feel it emotionally like a high-octane ping
in the pit of your stomach?

How do you get free of these emotions?
The painful or angry emotions
that come with the memory
will be gone when you truly forgive.

Are you willing
to take responsibility
and deal with what has happened
in your family tree?

Are you willing
to deal with what is happening spiritually
in your personal life?

Do you think it is possible
for God to change the genetic code
of disease in your family tree?

If you are engaged to be married,
are you both willing to look at your family tree
and deal with generational patterns
and your own personal sin?

Make a list
and follow the Ministry Prayer Model
in Appendix C.

Who are we going to for our healing?

God is our Creator. He is our Savior. He is our Healer. He is our Deliverer. He created us. Do we dare trust Him to know what's wrong with us? Would you, as His child, dare go to Him and ask Him to reveal to you the cause of your disease?

The fivefold ministry includes apostles, prophets, evangelists, pastors and teachers as gifts to the body.

> And he gave some, apostles; and some, prophets; and some, evangelists; and some, pastors and teachers;
> Ephesians 4:11

13. Has God ordained psychologists to be pastors?

yes _____ no _____

The medical community is not qualified to deal with spiritual issues. The church is ordained to deal with spiritual issues.

> To the intent that now unto the principalities and powers in heavenly places might be known by the church the manifold wisdom of God,
> Ephesians 3:10

Do you trust God when He says that He watches over His Word to perform it?

> Then said the Lord unto me, Thou hast well seen: for I will hasten my word to perform it.
> Jeremiah 1:12

God has created us with a free will. He is not going to force us:

- To come to Him.

- To become born again.

- To go to heaven.

You are going to have to respond to Him. Will you choose obedience or rebellion?

Are you willing to take responsibility for a spiritual root in exchange for healing? Would it be worth it? Would you dare believe that it could happen?

How does the immune system become compromised? The immune system becomes compromised because of fear and anxiety coming out of a broken heart. When you have a compromised immune system, you automatically have allergies.

> **A merry heart doeth good like a medicine:**
> **but a broken spirit drieth the bones.**
> Proverbs 17:22

14. Does this verse say that pesticides, smells and toxic chemicals destroy the immune system? No. It says a _____ _____ is what dries the bones and destroys the immune system. Is there someone in your life who broke your heart?

Blessings and Curses

Definition of Blessings and Curses

Blessing (Strong's Hebrew #1293) from Deuteronomy 28:2 means *benefit*. (See also root in Strong's Hebrew #1288)

Curses (Strong's Hebrew #7045) from Deuteronomy 28:15 means *vilification* or *abatement*. (See also root in Strong's Hebrew #7043)

Curse means the blessing (benefit) has been vilified or abated. Curse means an abatement or lessening of the blessing or benefit. Abatement means the standard has been decreased.

**A curse is anything
that is not full value of what is best for us.
It is important to understand
that curses do not come from God.**

Unforgiveness is an abatement of what forgiveness should look like. Are hemorrhoids an abatement or a benefit?

*Do you still have hemorrhoids?
How do you get free?*

*Give up anger and rage.
Be a "doer of the Word" according to James 1:23.*

Medical science says an angry person, statistically, has a higher chance of having a heart attack in the next two hours after anger. Is that an abatement or a benefit?

A blessing is a benefit that would be best for us. A curse is an abatement or a diminishing of the blessing or benefit.

Can a Christian have a curse?

Old Testament people did not understand evil and did not know there was a literal devil. This is not saying disease comes from God. They thought all things good and evil were from God. Only with Jesus, did more information come. Because *you* give yourself over to Satan, God *too* gives you over to Satan. Some do not believe Christians can have a "curse." Do Christians experience anything from the following list of "curses?"

> ··· if thou <u>will not hearken unto the voice </u>of the LORD thy God, to observe to do all his commandments, <u>all these curses shall come upon thee,</u> and overtake thee: Deuteronomy 28:15

List of Curses from Deuteronomy 28:15-68

Verse	KJV Translation	Strong's Definition	Application
MOSTLY BIOLOGICAL			
21	Pestilence	Destroying	Death from disease is a destroying plague.
22	Consumption	Emaciation	To emaciate, waste away, be thin, anemia, anorexia
22	Fever	Inflammation **root:** inflame	Fever under 103°, from inflammation, bacterial fever
22	Extreme burning	Fever (as hot) **root:** glow, melt, burn dry up	High fever, Burning fever over 103°
INCLUDING ANIMALS, PLANTS AND LAND			
22	Sword	Drought, cutting instrument (from its destructive effect) **root:** parch through drought, kill, destroy, desolate	Killing drought that parches the land, drought that cuts like a knife
22	Blasting	Blight **root:** scorch	Scorching blight, withering of plants
22	Mildew	Paleness **root:** vacuity of color, yellowish green of sickly vegetation	Sickly vegetation, loss of color or vitality

Verse	KJV Translation	Strong's Definition	Application
23	Heaven as brass	Copper **root:** red color	Out west drought and no rain produce dust-filled red skies.
23	Earth shall be iron	Firm, earth + wilderness	hard soil, heat parched soil
25	Flee from enemies seven different ways	This is opposite the blessing of our enemies fleeing from us seven different ways.	This is a fear issue. We are afraid of our enemies. (Mother-in-law?)
27	Botch	Inflammation, ulcer **root:** burn	To burn as with ulcers and boils
27	Emerods	Boil or ulcer **root:** burn	Hemorrhoids
27	Scab	Itching, scab, scurvy **root:** scratch	To scratch from itching, gum disease, scab[1], bleeding, scurvy (which is gum disease marked by spongy gums).

[1] Scab also means gum disease caused by lack of vitamin C. The gums bleed and make scabs. The ROOT behind this disease is: <u>You would not hear and obey</u>.

Verse	KJV Translation	Strong's Definition	Application
27	Itch	Itch, sum **root:** scrape	To scrape, itch, scratch, producing redness[2]
28	Madness	Craziness **root:** rave through insanity	Madness
28	Blindness	Blindness **root:** blind through film over the eyes	Not in touch with reality[3]
28	Astonishment of heart	Consternation	Double mindedness not knowing what to do[4]
29	Oppressed		Could also be depression. People who grope at noonday have no

[2] The Hebrew word for "itch" is found only this one time in the Bible. Anxiety produces an oversecretion of histamine in the skin. Doctors recommend topical antihistamine to treat this symptom.

[3] In the context of this verse the word blindness would be someone who has lost his reasoning. He is not in touch with reality, not able to process. This is talking about the ability to think. This is connected to the DSM-IV manual of psychiatric disease.

[4] Not knowing what to do, double mindedness, unstable in all his ways. (James 1:8, A double minded man is unstable in all his ways.) Heart can mean soul or spirit or combination of both. Here it is not psyche, just soul or mind. It could be confusion of understanding. *Webster's* consternation: strike down, dismay that hinders or throws someone into confusion.

Verse	KJV Translation	Strong's Definition	Application
			motivation
30	Betroth wife, another man lies with her		Divorce
30	Build a house, but not dwell there		Lose your house to foreclosure
30	Plant vineyard, another gathers		Lose your farm to foreclosure
34	Mad	Rave through insanity	Go raving insane
35	Lord smites in the knees		Disease of the knees
35	Sore botch cannot be healed	Sore: bad, evil **root:** spoil, make good for nothing Botch: inflammation **root:** burn	Bad, evil affliction, misery, calamity from sole of foot to top of head.[5] Botch = boil

---

[5] This affliction cannot be healed because they refuse to be a doer of the Word.

15. James 1:13 says,

> Let no man say when he is tempted, I am tempted of _____.

Deuteronomy says we choose a blessing or a curse by our obedience or disobedience.

> ²⁶Behold, I set before you this day a blessing and a curse;
> ²⁷A blessing, if ye obey the commandments of the Lord your God, which I command you this day:
> ²⁸And a curse, if ye will not obey the commandments of the Lord your God, but turn aside out of the way which I command you this day, to go after other gods, which ye have not known.
> ²⁹And it shall come to pass, when the Lord thy God hath brought thee in unto the land whither thou goest to possess it, that thou shalt put the blessing upon mount Gerizim, and the curse upon mount Ebal.   Deuteronomy 11:26-29

These scriptures are saying:

As God's people came into promise, they were immediately brought into a place of *discernment*. The discernment gave them a *choice* between good or evil.

You also must choose what you are going to believe and which path you will follow.

Here God is bringing a very powerful truth to His people.

He is saying: In obedience to Me and My commandments, the blessings (upon Mount Gerizim) are immediate and close by.

16. What does Mount Gerizim refer to? God's _____ _____ to obedience. page 74

However, "If you are disobedient, the curse (upon Mount Ebal) shall surely come." Mount Ebal is a symbol of the *delayed consequences* of disobedience.

In His grace and mercy, God has given us time for reflection and conviction.

17. The doctrine of Balaam teaches that you can keep your sin and still have _____.

In Deuteronomy 28, there are many blessings; then there are many curses. Under curses are *all manners of disease*, including other diseases "not written" will come upon you.

> Also every sickness, and every plague, which is not written in the book of this law, them will the Lord bring upon thee, until thou be destroyed.   Deuteronomy 28:61

18. Do you consider disease to be a blessing or a curse? _____

On the blessing side of Deuteronomy 28, is disease mentioned? No. Not one disease is mentioned.

Can you think of a disease that you would not consider a curse?

The Bible says when there is blessing, there is no disease, and when there is a curse, there is every manner of disease.

When we were freed from the power of sin and death at the cross, what did Christ say in John 19:30? He said, "It is finished."

If the penalty of the curse was paid, why do Christians have disease? Even though His broken body and His blood made our physical healing possible, we still have to appropriate what was done at the cross to be healed.

What did Christ do at the cross? He died for the sins of the world. His blood paid the price for all sins once and for all.

When He died, what was granted to us? His death granted us the right to appropriate the freedom that His work accomplished.

If His blood paid the price for all sins once and for all, why isn't everyone saved? Because each of us has to appropriate that work by faith.

Do we have to appropriate the finished work of Christ for healing as well? Yes. As it says in Isaiah 53:5, with His stripes we are healed. But you cannot get your freedom and still keep your sin.

Spiritually Rooted Disease is a Result of Separation on Three Levels

What are the three levels of separation that cause spiritually rooted disease?

19. Separation from _____. That includes His Word, His person and His love.

20. Separation from _____. Not accepting yourself. Allowing guilt and condemnation.

21. Separation from _____. This means having breaches in relationships.

The Power of the Tongue

We are either blessing or cursing with what we say. You are either building someone up or you are decreasing them.

> [8]The words of a talebearer are as wounds, and they go down into the innermost parts of the belly...
> [21]Death and life are in the power of the tongue: and they that love it shall eat the fruit thereof.   Proverbs 18: 8, 21

> And the tongue is a fire, a world of iniquity: so is the tongue among our members, that it defileth the whole body, and setteth on fire the course of nature; and it is set on fire of hell.
>   James 3:6

*Has anyone in your life
torn you down verbally?
Have you forgiven them?
Have you always built others up
by your words?*

Generational Blessings and Curses
Generational Sins and
Genetically Inherited Disease

And the seed of Israel separated themselves
from all strangers, and stood and confessed their
sins, and the iniquities of their fathers.

Nehemiah 9:2

22. Why did the children of captivity confess the sins
of their fathers? _____

The Family Tree of Abraham

Abraham was God's friend and the father of our
faith, but he had a spiritual problem. You can trace it as
it flows through his family tree. page 79

Abram lied about his wife Sarai because he was
afraid that her beauty would get him killed. In Genesis
12:11-12, Abram enticed his wife to lie, and he, himself,
lied to Pharaoh. (Abram's name was later changed to
Abraham.) He repented, but He did not learn the
lesson the first time. He did the same thing again a
second time in Genesis 20:2.

**The root problem behind people who lie
is fear of man, fear of rejection and fear of failure.
Primarily, it is from fear of man.**

The second generation manifested the same sin.
His son, Isaac, said word for word what his father
Abraham had said forty years before (Genesis 26). **Now a
second generation is operating in fear and lying, but
it did not end there.** Isaac's wife now knew how to lie,
and she collaborated with their son Jacob to deceive
him (Genesis 27).

**The third generation manifested the same sin
again.** Another generation of liars followed. Jacob's
son's lied to him regarding the matter of their brother,
Joseph. Jacob's wife Rachel lied to her father, Laban,
over the issue of idols (Genesis 31:35). In this generation
there are men *and* women *and* children lying.

That is where our faith begins — with a bunch of
fear-filled, lying saints.

**Abraham, believe it or not,
was called a "friend of God."**
(Isaiah 41:8, James 2:23)

**King David was called
a man after God's own heart.**

King David had a man murdered, stole his wife,
lusted, tempted Israel, but he was called a man after
God's own heart in Acts 13:22.

David's family was a tragedy: one son raped a
daughter, and another son rose up in sedition and
anarchy against him. One son died at childbirth
because of the sins of his father, David.

God holds the men responsible
for all matters of the family and the home.

The _male lineage_ traces ancestry through _his father_,
through his grandfather and his great-grandfather.

Do you have anything in common with your father,
grandfathers and great-grandfathers
that could be considered sin?

Did you have parents who did not know God?
You are a miracle if you know God now,
and your parents did not teach you about Him!

Do you know anything about your family tree
that is not right?

Did you ever hear rumors
about someone in your family tree?

The _female lineage_ traces ancestry back
through _her father_
and all the males before him.

The spiritual dynamics of the mother's family tree
travels from generation to generation
through the male (through her father).
That is why you can inherit things from your mother even
though they were in the family tree of her father.

What if there had been a man of God
in your home at some point?
At any point in the history of your family,
if there had been a man of God in the home,
he would have taken the necessary steps
to sanctify his wife and children.

Build your own family tree.

Were your family members Christians in past generations?

Were they righteous or unrighteous?

What were their personalities like?

Were they filled with fear, hate, envy, strife, etc.?

What did they do for a living?

Were they into alcohol, drugs and pornography?

*Did their lives contain
any of the elements that we are learning,
which are the roots for disease?*

*Go back as many generations as you can.
This will give you an idea
of what is in your family.*

*Every time you or anyone in your generations
stepped outside of the covenant of God,
your family tree was opened up
to the law and the penalty of the law.*

Does any incident come to your mind?

*If you have a genetically inherited disease, can you see the
spiritual root in your parents' lives?*

If sin is not dealt with before the Lord, you will pass it on to your seed.

Family Health
Tree Chart

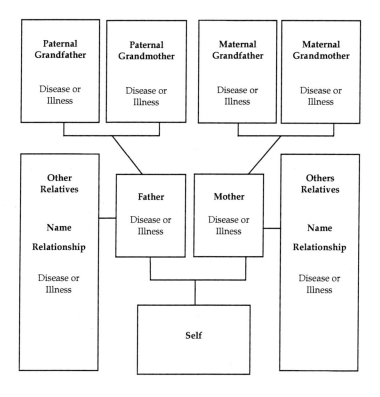

**It is good news that you are
in the new birth,
under the law of grace and mercy.
Under the old covenant,
you would be dead by sundown
for these sins.**

Generational Sins and Children

*Would you like to prevent disease in your children?
Wouldn't that be a more excellent way?*

Fear can be inherited. When a child has fear, or a disease rooted in fear, if you look back to the father and mother, and the grandfather and grandmother — on both sides of your family — you will find some kind of abuse, victimization or rejection. There will be someone who was not nurtured.

The Bible tells us in Ezekiel 18:19 that the children do not have to die for the sins of their fathers.

> **Yet say ye, Why? doth not the son bear the iniquity of the father? When the son hath done that which is lawful and right, and hath kept all my statutes, and hath done them, he shall surely live.** Ezekiel 18:19

How can the child get free? In cases where children have a disease or a problem resulting from a spiritual root that exists in a parent, we have seen *children* instantly healed of diseases when the *parent* came before God and resolved that sin issue.

God has made this provision for children that are not yet at the age of understanding.

What does the Bible say about children being sanctified by their parents?

> For the unbelieving husband is sanctified by the wife, and the unbelieving wife is sanctified by the husband: else were your children unclean; but now are they holy.
>
> 1 Corinthians 7:14

Healing Spiritually Rooted Diseases

How do you get healed from spiritually rooted disease?

All healing from spiritually rooted disease starts with coming back into alignment with God, His Word, His person, His nature, His precepts and what He planned on this planet for you from the beginning.

The solution is restoration.

How do you come back into alignment with God and get restored? You must first *accept yourself* in your relationship with God.

You must get rid of self-hatred.
You must get rid of self-bitterness and guilt
and come back in line with who you are
in the Father through Jesus Christ.

Can you love your neighbor without loving yourself? No. You cannot love your neighbor if you do not love yourself. It is not possible.

*First bring the strength of God
into your life.
Then bring the strength of God
into others' lives, in that order.*

Prolonged breakdown in the above sequence produces many, many diseases. Why? Because God commanded that you shall love your neighbor as yourself.

**If you see a disease, you see a curse.
If you see a curse, there is a reason for it.**

As the bird by wandering, as the swallow by flying, so the curse causeless shall not come.

Proverbs 26:2

If...you see a disease ...
Then...you know there is a cause ...
But... you can repent, and remove the cause.

23.   What has to be removed? _____

Removing the spiritual root is called *sanctification*. God has called us to be a people who are *sanctified without spot or blemish* (Ephesians 5:27).

What has He called you to?
He has called you to holiness.
He has called you to walk before Him
because He is your God.
He has called you to be cleansed...
perfecting holiness in the fear of God.
(2 Corinthians 7:1)

The Chastening of the Lord

The Bible tells us that when we follow our enemies, God gives us over to the blessings of our enemies.

What are the enemy's blessings? The enemy's blessings are *curses*. The blessings of their enemies were *oppression* and *bondage* (Deuteronomy 28:15).

> But it shall come to pass, if thou wilt not hearken unto the voice of the LORD thy God, to observe to do all his commandments and his statutes which I command thee this day; that all these curses shall come upon thee, and overtake thee: Deuteronomy 28:15

When the Old Testament saints had finally "had enough," what did they do? They cried out to God in repentance.

How would God respond? He would end their captivity, and He would bless them. He would release them when they repented and turned back to Him. Keep this in mind: the Lord is not putting evil on us, but giving us over to the devices of our own heart until we have "had enough."

What happens when we recognize the spiritual defects of our life through conviction by the Holy Spirit and through the washing of the Word?

When we do these things, the spiritual defect is then *purified*.

The Baptism of Fire is the purging work, the sanctifying work of the Holy Spirit.

How do we know that God did not give the spiritual defect? That would be contrary to His holy nature.

> Let no man say when he is tempted, I am tempted of God: for God cannot be tempted with evil, neither tempteth he any man.
>
> James 1:13

What is His desire for us regarding the spiritual defect? He wants to purge it from us.

> He that committeth sin is of the devil; for the devil sinneth from the beginning. For this purpose the Son of God was manifested, that he might destroy the works of the devil.   1 John 3:8

> How God anointed Jesus of Nazareth with the Holy Ghost and with power: who went about doing good, and healing all that were oppressed of the devil; for God was with him.
>
> Acts 10:38

*If you see something in your life
that you thought was
"just the way you are,"
but you now realize that it is sin,
turn to the section on the 8 Rs
and apply the study.*

Answers to Unit Two

1. Father

2. Son

3. Holy Spirit

4. the Father

5. Father

6. Father

7. Father

8. Father

9. Father

10. Father

11. guilt

12. autoimmune

13. no

14. broken spirit

15. God

16. quick response

17. blessings

18. curse

19. God

20. self

21. others

22. They were the product of their father's disobedience and saw the same sins in their own lives and the lives of their children.

23. You must get the spiritual root removed.

Study Unit Three:
Bitterness

See *A More Excellent Way*™, 7th Edition, pages 95-100*

Bitterness is a strongman in Satan's kingdom that produces intense ill will or even hatred in a person under its influence. Seven lesser yet increasingly more evil spirits we call "underlings" are the fruit of bitterness and act as armor to protect or hide bitterness.

We must recognize that bitterness and its underling spirits want to separate you from God and from His peace. They will separate you from peace with yourself and with others. When others violate us, we sometimes get into conflict with them because we make them evil along with the evil they did. Do you know the problem this creates? Sin is our enemy, not them!

> **For we wrestle not against flesh and blood, but against principalities, against powers, against the rulers of the darkness of this world, against spiritual wickedness in high places.**
> Ephesians 6:12

God did not create you from the foundation of the world as a sinner. He created you as a saint and as His son or daughter forever.

Bitterness is a principality that depends on the seven spirits under it as armor to hold it in place.

---

* Page numbers refer to *A More Excellent Way*™

1. List the seven (underling) spirits of bitterness.

   a. _____

   b. _____

   c. _____

   d. _____

   e. _____

   f. _____

   g. _____

Unforgiveness

2. Hebrews 12:15 says,
   > Looking diligently lest any man fail of
   > the grace of God; lest any root of bitterness
   > springing up _____ you, and
   > thereby many be defiled.

**Unforgiveness keeps a record of wrongs.
It can come into your life
because of injury done to you by someone else.**

If you still remember what your aunt did to you
many years ago, and you still do not like her, you have
unforgiveness. Unforgiveness keeps a record of wrongs
and causes another dimension of spiritual dynamics
called resentment.

Resentment

3. Resentment is the record of wrongs that you are
   _____ onto and meditating on.

4. When you think about your aunt in your head,
   AND you feel her in your heart (or belly, meaning

in your spirit), you have resentment. It is a spiritual problem that separates us from other people, and it is the foundation of future fear such as: fear of _____, fear of _____, fear of failure, etc.

Retaliation

5.   Retaliation wants to ____ _____. After resentment simmers within us, we think about ways to get back at people, to make them pay for what they did to us.

Anger

6.   After unforgiveness, resentment and retaliation have been building within us, then comes anger. Anger reminds you that you have not forgiven them, that you still resent them and want to get even with them. You have crossed a line because the first three spirits can be hidden, but anger is vocalized.   You can see anger in a person's _____ and hear it in their _____.

Hatred

7.   After anger and wrath gain a foothold, then comes hatred.   Hatred begins to develop the _____ modality. Anger starts to vocalize; hatred starts to eliminate.

Violence

8.   Violence does _____ damage to the other person.

Murder

9.   Murder is the elimination of a person on all levels. It can be physical murder or murder with the _____, which is character assassination.

Forgive 70 x 7

Forgiveness is What God Expects of Us – 70 x 7.

> **Jesus saith unto him, I say not unto thee, Until seven times: but, Until seventy times seven.** Matthew 18:22

The Lord gave Pastor Henry understanding of 70 x 7. There are three eight-hour segments in a day: Eight for work, eight for family and eight for sleep.

10.   With sixty minutes in each hour, eight hours x 60 minutes per hour equals _____.

11.   Comparing, 70 x 7 equals _____.

The point is that 490, the number of times to forgive, is more than 480, the number of minutes in each section of our day. So minute by minute, hour by hour, day by day we are to forgive and release those who defile us.

12.   Forgiving another person does not mean _____ their sin.

We are not to take another person's sin into our body!

13. What is our job when people defile us?

_____

We are to judge ourselves, not judge others.

But why dost thou judge thy brother? or why dost thou set at nought thy brother? for we shall all stand before the judgment seat of Christ.
Romans 14:10

14. How can you prepare yourself now for any potential future bitterness people may have against you? _____

Bitterness and its underling spirits come into our lives in different ways.

They can be inherited as a familiar spirit passed down from generation to generation.

They can be acquired due to expectations of others not being fulfilled and our going into bitterness as a result.

They can be acquired due to circumstances in life and our choosing to respond with bitterness.

They can be modeled to us and we become programmed to allow these spirits to work out their evil nature through us.

We can have a personality of bitterness as a result of not being able to separate ourselves from bitterness.

Can you recognize any of the underlings of bitterness
as you examine your relationships?

Are you having flashbacks
of things done to you in the past?
Are you keeping a record of wrongs?
Do you want to get even?

When you think of a certain person,
do you feel resentment or anger?

Do you hate someone?
Have you committed murder,
including murder in your heart or your tongue?

Have you developed any bitterness toward God?
Do you blame God for evil in the world or in your life?
Have you become angry and rebelled against God
because someone has hurt you and now you blame God?
Have you become disappointed or angry
when God did not answer your prayers
the way you thought He should?

Are you willing to come out of agreement with bitterness
and any of the underlings by choosing to obey God's Word?

If you will practice sanctification by doing the 8 Rs,
you can restore peace with God,
with yourself,
and with others in your life.

Answers to Unit Three

1. a. unforgiveness b. resentment
    c. retaliation d. anger e. hatred
    f. violence g. murder (which includes
    murder with the tongue)

2. trouble

3. holding

4. man, rejection

5. get even

6. strong feeling, voice

7. elimination

8. painful

9. tongue

10. 480

11. 490

12. condoning

13. release them, get back before God, get our
    heart right with God, and keep on going

14. separate them from their sin, by choosing
    to have a heart of forgiveness towards
    them in advance and by seeing them and
    myself through God's eyes

Study Unit Four:
Separation

See *A More Excellent Way*™, 7th Edition, pages 101-114*

Separation is the first step toward appropriating the freedom and deliverance promised to us as believers.

Separation means separating yourself
from the sin that lives within you
and separating others
from the sin that lives within them.

Separation is where true forgiveness begins. It is where the healing of hearts, minds, bodies and relationships can begin.

1.   Separation is the beginning of _____.

In Romans 7:14-15, Paul is speaking about himself. He has been a believer and an apostle for at least 20 years. He's talking about his life and his challenges in living a Christian life.

> ¹⁴For we know that the law is spiritual: but I am carnal, sold under sin.
> ¹⁵For that which I do I allow not: for what I would, that do I not; but what I hate, that do I.
> Romans 7:14-15

---

* Page numbers refer to *A More Excellent Way*™

Does that sound familiar?
Do you ever want to do things that you are not doing?
Do you ever do the things that you hate?
Do you think Paul was sinless?

Only one man was sinless, the man Christ Jesus.

The rest of us are sinners, saved by grace, and working out our salvation *daily* with fear and trembling.

> Wherefore, my beloved, as ye have always obeyed, not as in my presence only, but now much more in my absence, work out your own salvation with fear and trembling.
>
> Philippians 2:12

2. Psalm 95:7 says,

> For he is our God; and we are the people of his pasture, and the sheep of his hand, _____ if ye will hear his voice.

3. Scripture says in 2 Corinthians 6:2,

> For he saith, I have heard thee in a time accepted, and in the day of salvation have I succoured thee: behold, _____ is the accepted time; behold, _____ is the day of salvation.

4. Luke 9:23 says,

> And he said to them all, If any man will come after me, let him deny himself, and take up his cross _____, and follow me.

5. Philippians 2:12 says,

> Wherefore, my beloved, as ye have always obeyed, not as in my presence only, but _____ much more in my absence, work out your own salvation with fear and trembling.
>
> If then I do that which I would not, I consent unto the law that it is good.   Romans 7:16

Paul is saying, (paraphrase) if I do those things that are evil, I am telling the law, or the Word, that this new law that I am following (which represents evil) is good, and the Word of God is evil.

6. Are we sometimes following a "different law" in our lives than the law of God? yes _____ no _____

7. When the Word says, *Forgive your brother*, and we do not, are we following a different law, a different gospel, and a different way of thinking?

yes _____ no_____

Paul is saying that when he does those evil things he wishes he would not do, he's consenting unto the law of God, that this thing that he should not be doing is good, and that automatically puts him under the authority of another gospel. When we hate our brother, we are affirming a new gospel that overthrows the gospel of our God.

Think about the people
who have injured you in your lifetime,
either through word or deed.
Think about people who did not treat you right,
victimized you, lied about you, or abused you
either emotionally, physically, verbally,
or maybe even sexually.

When you think of their name, or their face,
whether they are living or dead,
what do you feel?
Do you have that high-octane ping going off inside?

Is there anyone in your life that you resent or even hate?
Is there anyone that you need to forgive?
Do you need to forgive yourself?

If so, turn to A More Excellent Way™, 7th Edition, Appendix C
and go through Walk Out.

IT IS VERY IMPORTANT for you to understand that sin involves the overthrowing of the government, the laws and the precepts of God.

By sinning, we are establishing another gospel in the earth for mankind to follow to their destruction, not to their benefit. We do not like to think that we have sin in our lives as Christians, BUT—

When we allow fear to rule our lives, we are affirming and agreeing with the gospel of fear. Fear destroys faith, which is of God.

8. When we allow guilt to rule our lives, we are affirming the gospel of _____ to the destruction of _____ by God. page 102

Daily,
we are establishing
one gospel or another.

9. We are either establishing the law of the kingdom of _____ or we are establishing the law of _____'s kingdom. page 102

You cannot serve two masters; either you are going to love the one or hate the other (Matthew 6:24). That has to be understood with regard to certain diseases before you can be healed.

You cannot be healed of an autoimmune disease
and hang onto self-hatred.
Which kingdom do you choose to establish
in your life today?

We are working out our own salvation daily by faith through grace and mercy. This is the work of *sanctification*. Paul is describing himself, and he's not been cleaned up yet. Neither have you. If you tell me you are sinless, the Word says whosoever says he has not sinned is a liar. These scriptures are addressed to believers who sin after conversion.

10. Scripture says in 1 John 1:10,
    If we say that we have _____ _____, we make him a liar, and his word is not in us.

Error in the church

Some teach that if you sinned after conversion, you were never saved. Does that mean there are no Christians in the earth today because we all fall short of the glory of God, every day?

> For all have sinned, and come short of the glory of God; Romans 3:23

While many say this scripture applies only to unbelievers, a look at Christians will reveal many of the same sins in both the saved and unsaved. Both have fallen short of the glory of God, and both need to repent.

11. Would God require the unsaved to repent for a sin and not require the saved to repent of that sin?

yes _____ no _____

Scripture refutes the position that Romans 3:23 applies only to unbelievers.

> ¹What shall we say then? Shall we continue in sin, that grace may abound?
> ²God forbid. How shall we, that are dead to sin, live any longer therein? Romans 6:1-2

Have you ever struggled with any insecurities and fears?
Paul, in Romans 7:17, is talking about
when he is doing things that are not right.

Paul was an apostle, born again,
filled with the Spirit of God, teaching righteousness,
and he's saying he has sin within.

Paul also needed ministry!
If Paul needed help, what is our condition?

The sin within us is talking to us in our minds, trying to cause us to commit a sin – any sin. Remember sin is not just robbing a bank; it is also resenting our neighbor. Study the Seven Steps to Sin in Appendix B in *A More Excellent Way*™, 7th Edition.

**We must separate ourselves
from the sin that dwells within us
and from the sin that dwells within our neighbor.**

12. When you look at your neighbor, you are going to have to be able to _____ them from their sin.

**Our battle is not with flesh and blood
but with entities from another kingdom.**

For we wrestle not against flesh and blood, but against principalities, against powers, against the rulers of the darkness of this world, against spiritual wickedness in high *places*.
Ephesians 6:12

The Word of God is making manifest those creatures that are within. These are the "yucky-puckies," those "crispy critters" that Paul is talking about in Romans 7. Dealing with this stuff, receiving healing and deliverance from those things that dwell within, is the process of *sanctification*. This is in the realm of the spirit.

**Receiving healing and deliverance
from those things that dwell within
is the process of sanctification.**

13. Are medical doctors trained to deal with the spiritual roots of disease? yes ___ no ___

**I cannot forgive my brother unless I practice separation.
I cannot forgive myself unless I practice separation.**

When people victimize me, I am able to see the evil in them (which now controls them) that is now making a victim of me. I can see it is not them. It is the sin that lives within them. So I can exchange compassion for bitterness according to the knowledge of God.

*Did you realize that in Galatians 5:19-21,
strife is found in the same verses:*

*As murder?
As adultery?
As fornication?*

¹⁹Now the works of the flesh are manifest, which are *these*; <u>Adultery,</u> fornication, uncleanness, lasciviousness,

²⁰Idolatry, witchcraft, hatred, variance, emulations, wrath, <u>strife,</u> seditions, heresies,

²¹Envyings, <u>murders,</u> drunkenness, revellings, and such like: of the which I tell you before, as I have also told *you* in time past, that

they which do such things shall not inherit the
kingdom of God.   Galatians 5:19-21

All these evil things come from within, and
defile the man.   Mark 7:23

14. According to Mark 7:23, where do all these evil
things (i.e., things that defile a man) come from?

_____

Romans 1:28-31, Mark 7 and Galatians 5 list many
sins. We see these at one level or another in ourselves
and others. In reviewing the sins, you will note that
there are no white lies or even big or little sins. There is
just sin and we need to separate ourselves from it and
deal with it.

15. Why is that? It is because we are not _____.
page 106

These same sins are the root causes of our
biological, spiritual and mental diseases.

**The day that I learned
to separate myself from my sin
is the day that sanctification
began in my life.**

¹⁸For I know that in me (that is, in my flesh,)
dwelleth no good thing: for to will is present
with me; but _how_ to perform that which is good
I find not.
¹⁹For the good that I would I do not: but the
evil which I would not, that I do.
²⁰Now if I do that I would not, it is no more I
that do it, but sin that dwelleth in me.
          Romans 7:18-20

Have you ever found yourself viewing sin like Paul?

*Have you ever had a wonderful heart toward God,
and the harder you tried the behinder you got?*

*Have you ever had struggles in your Christian walk,
where it just did not come together
as fast as you wanted it to?*

*You look into the mirror of the Bible,
and when you turn away, do you see the sin?*

*That is what Paul is seeing with the eyes of honesty.
Do not forget what you saw in the perfect law of liberty.
That is the real you.*

Paul says more than once that it is not him that is doing what he does not want to do, but it is sin that is dwelling in him.

16. Do you think he was recognizing his own need for deliverance? yes ___ no ___

**The beginning of understanding
is being able to separate yourself
from the sin that dwells within,
that is acting out its nature through you.**

This is the full meaning of Hebrews 4:12-13.

> [12]For the word of God is quick, and powerful, and sharper than any two-edged sword, piercing even to the dividing asunder of soul and spirit, and of the joints and marrow, and is a discerner of the thoughts and intents of the heart.
> [13] Neither is there any creature that is not manifest in his sight: but all things are naked

and opened unto the eyes of him with whom we
have to do.   Hebrews 4:12-13

The sin that dwells within (Romans 7:18-20) that
Paul talks about is identified in Hebrews 4:13 as the
creatures that need to be made open and naked before
Him with whom we have to do.

This is the beginning of healing.

There is therefore now no condemnation to
them which are in Christ Jesus, who walk not
after the flesh, but after the Spirit.   Romans 8:1

Condemnation occurs because the only place that
you are free from condemnation under the law is when
you are walking after the Spirit of God. When you step
outside those parameters, you are back under the law
again, and there is a consequence. Your freedom is
directly related to your obedience.

See *A More Excellent Way*™, 7th edition, page 109 and Deuteronomy chapter 28 in
KJV Bible.

There is a consequence
to sin and disobedience
to God's Word.

That is not legalism; that is simply what Jesus
meant when He said,

If ye love me, keep my commandments.
                                   John 14:15

Keeping God's commandments is not legalism.
Taking God's commandments and forcing them down
someone's throat is legalism.

> Who also hath made us able ministers of the
> new testament; not of the letter, but of the spirit:
> for the letter killeth, but the spirit giveth life.
> 2 Corinthians 3:6

Paul is dealing with an issue.

> But I see another law in my members,
> warring against the law of my mind, and
> bringing me into captivity to the law of sin
> which is in my members.   Romans 7:23

He's saying, I myself serve the law of God, but I have a problem in my life. I have sin that dwells within me.

Fear is sin. Unforgiveness is sin. Strife is sin. Self-hatred is sin. Heresy is sin. Adultery is sin. Lasciviousness is sin. Gossip is sin. Backbiting is sin. Causing church splits is sin. Jealousy and envy are sin.

It is not what goes in your mouth that defiles you; it is what comes from *within* you, out of your mouth.

> Not that which goeth into the mouth defileth
> a man; but that which cometh out of the mouth,
> this defileth a man.   Matthew 15:11

Paul is addressing the believer, not the unbeliever, in 2 Corinthians 7:1. Very clearly, Paul is setting the stage for something called sanctification subsequent to salvation.

Sanctification is the process that takes place when we get before God and take an honest look at ourselves, when we survey our past generations and deal with the sin we find in ourselves and in our generations. It is coming before God to let Him "work us over." One result of repenting for, and removing the sin in our lives is that spiritual, biological and psychological diseases are also removed. (Refer to the Family Health Tree in Unit Two for assistance in examining family diseases and spiritual roots.)

The Lord is saying to you today:
I am here knocking.
Would you open the door of your heart?
Would you let Me come in with the Holy Spirit
and cleanse you, sanctify you,
and remove the things
that are separating you from Me?

Would you let Me
heal you? deliver you?

Know ye not, that to whom ye yield yourselves servants to obey, his servants ye are to whom ye obey; whether of sin unto death, or of obedience unto righteousness? Romans 6:16

In conclusion, in Romans 6:16 listed above, the big question is this:

Who is your master?
What are you a servant to?
Sin unto death
or obedience unto righteousness?

If you decide to serve sin, then sin becomes your lord, and you become its slave. Has the body of sin been destroyed in your life or are you still serving sin today?

Romans 8:1

One of the tragedies of Bible translations is the removal of one half of Romans 8:1. In removing the second part of Romans 8:1, the conditions of not being condemned in Christ Jesus have been removed.

There is therefore now no condemnation to them which are in Christ Jesus, who walk not after the flesh, but after the Spirit.   Romans 8:1

Those who continue to walk after the flesh bring themselves back into condemnation, and Satan has a legal right to their life until they repent.

The fruit of our service to sin is spiritual, psychological and biological disease.

Answers to Unit Four

1. healing

2. today

3. now, now

4. daily

5. now

6. yes

7. yes

8. guilt, forgiveness

9. God, Satan (or vice versa)

10. not sinned

11. No, that would make Him unjust.

12. separate

13. no

14. within

15. sanctified

16. Yes, he's looking at himself with eyes of honesty.

Study Unit Five:
The 8 Rs to Freedom
See *A More Excellent Way*™, 7th Edition, pages 115 – 122*

Pathway to Wholeness

Our Pathway **to Wholeness and Freedom** is a daily journey. The **8 Rs** are signposts along that journey. Each **R** represents a choice or a step into receiving or keeping our freedom. Many testimonies of freedom have come to this ministry from people who read this book and applied the **8 Rs**.

List the **8 Rs**.

1. _____

2. _____

3. _____

4. _____

5. _____

6. _____

7. _____

8. _____

* Page numbers refer to *A More Excellent Way*™

Recognize

You must recognize what it is.

Definition of RECOGNIZE: To acknowledge formally, to admit, to perceive clearly (*Merriam-Webster's Collegiate Dictionary*, 10th Edition)

9. According to Isaiah 5:13, who has no knowledge and has gone into captivity? _____

> Therefore my people are gone into captivity, because they have no knowledge: and their honourable men are famished, and their multitude dried up with thirst.   Isaiah 5:13

10. According to Hosea 4:6, who has no knowledge and is destroyed? _____

> My people are destroyed for lack of knowledge: because thou hast rejected knowledge, I will also reject thee, that thou shalt be no priest to me: seeing thou hast forgotten the law of thy God, I will also forget thy children.
> Hosea 4:6

11. Hebrews 5:14 instructs us to practice having our _____ exercised to _____ BOTH _____ and _____.

> But strong meat belongeth to them that are of full age, even those who by reason of use have their senses exercised to discern both good and evil.   Hebrews 5:14

How do I recognize the problem?
(Have discernment.)

How do I get discernment?
(Ask for it and get knowledge.)

Make a list of what you recognize (discern)
that is not of God in yourself.

Responsibility

You must take responsibility
for what you recognize.

Definition of RESPONSIBILITY: Accountability
(*Merriam-Webster's Collegiate Dictionary*, 10th Edition)

If you think "That's just the way I am," then do you need to take responsibility for:

bitterness?	envy or jealousy?	fear?
unforgiveness?	criticism?	rejection?
resentment?	accusations?	self-hatred?
anger?	occultism?	rebellion?

The scripture says we are being changed into the image of the Lord. In Unit One we learned that sanctification is a PROCESS. In Appendix C we learn about Walking Out to Wholeness.

> **But we all, with open face beholding as in a glass the glory of the Lord, are changed into the same image from glory to glory, even as by the Spirit of the Lord.** 2 Corinthians 3:18

12. From glory to glory we are being _____

Someone
is going to have to get spiritual.

13. Do you think the other person needs to get spiritual first, or do you need to get spiritual first? _____

How do I take responsibility?
(Make the decision to do the right thing.)

Change without expecting
the other person to change.

Apply the principles
of the teaching on Separation
and separate those
who have hurt you
from their sin.

Psalm 51:3-4 is a scriptural example of taking responsibility for our actions. David committed sexual sin and murder, and realized that he also sinned against God. He recognized his sin and took responsibility.

> [3]For I acknowledge my transgressions: and my sin is ever before me.
> [4]Against thee, thee only, have I sinned, and done this evil in thy sight: that thou mightest be justified when thou speakest, and be clear when thou judgest.   Psalm 51:3-4

Repent

Repent to God for participating with what you recognize.

Definition of REPENT: Think differently (Strong's Greek # 3340)

Definition of REPENT from *Merriam-Webster's Collegiate Dictionary, 10th Edition*: To turn from sin and dedicate oneself to the amendment of one's life; to feel sorrow, regret or contrition.

Scripture instructs us to repent for our sins and turn away from them.

> Therefore I will judge you, O house of Israel, every one according to his ways, saith the Lord God. Repent, and turn yourselves from all your transgressions; so iniquity shall not be your ruin. Ezekiel 18:30

14. Scripture says in 1 John 1:9,
> If we _____ our sins, he is faithful and just to forgive us our sins, and to cleanse us from all unrighteousness.

From the list you just made
of what you recognize in yourself that is not of God,
are you willing to repent for these things?

Refer to the model prayer in Appendix C on Walk Out.

Renounce

Make what you recognize your enemy and renounce it.

Definition of RENOUNCE: To refuse to follow further (*Merriam-Webster's Collegiate Dictionary*, 10th Edition)

To renounce literally means to "turn away from." Develop a perfect hatred for evil in your life. (Pastor Donna Wright says we need to at least begin to WANT to develop a perfect hatred for evil in our life. When we participate with "rejection," we do not hate "rejection.")

Renounce what you have just repented for and tell it to go. Tell it out loud so it can hear your voice. It cannot read your mind, but it can hear your voice. You must fall out of agreement with sin by renouncing it.

Many people repent, but they really do not mean it. They do not have remorse; they do not change on the inside. Other people repent but they do not renounce, so repentance becomes an exercise in recycling!

An example of renouncing follows. Note that it is spoken out loud, with conviction. Let your declarations be made boldly that all things both visible and invisible may know the intent of your confession.

Speak so that everything
visible and invisible
can know your intention.

You say to fear, you say to bitterness,
"Listen to my voice.
I renounce everything you stand for in my life."

And say more (as the Spirit leads you).

Editor's Note: See Appendix E-9 in *A More Excellent Way*™, 7th Edition for Testimony of Healing of Sleep Apnea and Use of "Renouncing" to keep the healing.

Remove it

Get rid of it once and for all

Definition of REMOVE: Get rid of, eliminate (*Merriam-Webster's Collegiate Dictionary*, 10th Edition)

Removing sin is this: "Not only do I renounce you, but you and I cannot exist at the same place at the same time together. I am removing you; you have to go." The Bible never teaches you to cohabit with an enemy. It teaches that you identify the darkness and remove it.

> Cast away from you all your transgressions, whereby ye have transgressed; and make you a new heart and a new spirit: for why will ye die, O house of Israel?   Ezekiel 18:31

15.   According to this scripture what are you to do with what you have recognized, taken responsibility for, repented for and renounced?

Cohabitation with the enemy is strictly forbidden.

Remove means
breaking the power of that sin in your life
and casting it out.

Remove means
not hanging out with self-rejection
or bitterness anymore.

Remove means
not hanging out with those people
who might lure you back to that sin!

Refer to Prayer of Deliverance in Appendix C on Walk Out.

Resist

When it tries to come back, resist it.

Definition of RESIST: Take a stand, exert oneself as to counteract or defeat (*Merriam-Webster's Collegiate Dictionary*, 10th Edition)

Scripture says the devil will flee from us if we resist him.

Submit yourselves therefore to God. Resist
the devil, and he will flee from you.   James 4:7

16. Before we can resist the devil we must
_____ ___ _____.

> When the unclean spirit is gone out of a man, he walketh through dry places, seeking rest; and finding none, he saith, I will return unto my house whence I came out.   Luke 11:24

What you have dealt with will try to come back!

To resist it and keep it from coming back, you must submit to God.

How do you submit yourself to God? Recognize the indwelling presence of sin, take responsibility for it, repent for it, renounce it, remove it and resist it.

<u>Draw nigh to God.</u>

If God says you have not been given the spirit of fear, then <u>believe it!</u>

17. Scripture says in 2 Timothy 1:7,
> For God hath not given us the spirit of fear; but of _____, and of _____, and of a _____ _____.

If God said you are to forgive your brother, then forgive your brother whether you feel like it or not. That is drawing nigh to God.

When you have dealt with it, you will still remember what your brother did to you in 1942, but you will no longer feel him in the pit of your stomach, because you have been delivered.

Rejoice

Give God thanks for setting you free.

Definition of REJOICE: To feel joy or great delight (*Merriam-Webster's Collegiate Dictionary*, 10th Edition)

In the Old Testament, read Isaiah 35:1-10. page 120

In the New Testament it says,

> **Rejoice in the Lord alway: and again I say, Rejoice.** Philippians 4:4

Give glory to God for your freedom!

Make a list of what you have to rejoice over.

Make a list of what God has done for you.

Make a list of what God has done for others.

Restore

Help someone else get free.

Definition of RESTORE: To renew, give back (*Merriam-Webster's Collegiate Dictionary*, 10th Edition)

Part of restoring is bringing the gospel to those you love, instructing those sinners that are separated from the refreshing of the Lord and discipling them.

In the Old Testament read Isaiah 58:1-12. page 121

18. Galatians 6:1-3 says,

> ¹Brethren, if a man be overtaken in a fault, ye which are spiritual, _____ such an one in the spirit of meekness; considering thyself, lest thou also be tempted.
> ²Bear ye one another's burdens, and so fulfil the law of Christ.
> ³For if a man think himself to be something, when he is nothing, he deceiveth himself.

First Corinthians says,

> ²⁵That there should be no schism in the body; but that the members should have the same care one for another.
> ²⁶And whether one member suffer, all the members suffer with it; or one member be honoured, all the members rejoice with it.
> 1 Corinthians 12:25-26

Answers to Unit Five

1.   Recognize

2.   Responsibility

3.   Repent

4.   Renounce

5.   Remove

6.   Resist

7.   Rejoice

8.   Restore

9.   God's people

10. God's people

11. senses, discern, good, evil

12. changed

13. I need to get spiritual.

14. confess our sins

15. remove it

16. submit to God

17. power, love, sound mind

18. restore

Study Unit Six:
Gifts of the Spirit

See *A More Excellent Way*™, 7th Edition, pages 123–126*

God can and does deliver and heal people today. The evidence is overwhelming that this is true. In order to meet the need for establishing teams across America to teach churches how to heal the sick and to cast out devils, members of the church must recognize the benefits of the fivefold ministry and gifts of the Spirit in order to help God's people gain their health and freedom.

The Fivefold Ministry

In Ephesians 4:11-12, there is clear evidence that the fivefold ministry has been established by Jesus Christ to equip the saints for service. As a member of the body of Christ, you are equipped to do the same works that Jesus did and even greater.

> ¹¹And he gave some, apostles; and some, prophets; and some, evangelists; and some, pastors and teachers;
> ¹²For the perfecting of the saints, for the work of the ministry, for the edifying of the body of Christ: Ephesians 4:11-12

> ²⁷Now ye are the body of Christ, and members in particular.
> ²⁸And God hath set some in the church, first apostles, secondarily prophets, thirdly teachers, after that miracles, then gifts of healings, helps, governments, diversities of tongues.

---

* Page numbers refer to *A More Excellent Way*™

> [29]Are all apostles? are all prophets? are all teachers? are all workers of miracles?
> [30]Have all the gifts of healing? do all speak with tongues? do all interpret?
>
> 1 Corinthians 12:27-30

First Corinthians 12:27-30 gives the foundational teaching to support God's plan for the equipping of the saints for the profit of the body of Christ. God has set these things in the church.

1. Are all apostles?   yes____ no ____
2. Are some apostles?   yes____ no ____
3. Are all prophets?   yes____ no ____
4. Are some prophets?   yes____ no ____
5. Are all teachers?   yes____ no ____
6. Are some teachers?   yes____ no ____
7. Are all workers of miracles?   yes____ no ____
8. Are some workers of miracles?   yes____ no____
9. Do all have the gifts of healing?   yes____ no ____
10. Do some have the gifts of healing?   yes____ no ____
11. Do all speak with tongues?   yes____ no ____
12. Do some speak with tongues?   yes____ no ____
13. Do all interpret?   yes____ no ____
14. Do some interpret?   yes____ no ____

You are part of the body of Christ and members in particular!

19. Name the gifts in 1 Corinthians 12:27-30.

a. _____

b. _____

c. _____

d. _____

e. _____

f. _____

g. _____

h. _____

*Do you recognize that His gifts
have operated in your life?*

*Make a list of the gifts
given to you by the Spirit.*

*OR do you depend on others
to be used of God in this way?*

*According to 1 Corinthians 12,
the body is to take care of the body.*

*Does the Holy Spirit only use <u>others</u>
to operate in and through?*

*Are <u>you</u> available
to be a blessing and encouragement
to others?*

The gifts of the Spirit have been given for use in and by the church. These gifts were given to bring you to a place of health. For example, the gift of healing is a gift available from God to stop the forward motion of disease and bring the power of God in so that the body will heal. But if an evil spirit has a hold on your life, then the gift of discerning of spirits can help evict those evil spirits from your life. These gifts were given to benefit you.

Three dimensions of physical healing

There are three dimensions of physical healing.

- The healing of body tissue
- The regeneration of body tissue
- The removal of things that are alien to us spiritually (spiritual roots)

God receives no glory from your disease. In fact, healing is something called greater grace. (See Study Unit Nine for more discussion on greater grace.)

Conclusion

We need saints ministering one to another under the oversight of the fivefold ministry. The body is to take care of the body in all matters of health and sanity.

> ...the manifestation (of each of the gifts) of the Spirit is given to every man to profit withal.
> 1 Corinthians 12:7

The healing of disease is for the glory of God!

Answers to Unit Six

1. no

2. yes

3. no

4. yes

5. no

6. yes

7. no

8. yes

9. no

10. yes

11. no

12. yes

13. no

14. yes

15. a. apostles   b. prophets   c. teachers
    d. miracles   e. gifts of healings   f. helps
    g. governments h. diversities of tongues

Study Unit Seven:
Fear, Stress and Physiology

See *A More Excellent Way*™, 7th Edition, pages 127–170*

Physiology of Multiple Chemical Sensitivities/Environmental Illness (MCS/EI)

Many people with MCS/EI are universal reactors. That means they react (allergically) to almost everything.

When Pastor Henry Wright was first asked for help with the healing of MCS/EI, the Holy Spirit led him to Proverbs 17:22, which gave him the understanding that part of the immune system is in the marrow of the bones.

> **A merry heart doeth good like a medicine:
> but a broken spirit drieth the bones.**
>
> Proverbs 17:22

Fear, Anxiety and Stress Affect Your Life

1. The immune system becomes compromised and then destroyed. In Proverbs 17:22, we learn the immune system (marrow of the bone) is destroyed by a _____ _____.

---

* Page numbers refer to *A More Excellent Way*™

2.   Sometimes the female gets sick more often because she is more susceptible to spiritual and emotional damage that has come to her in her life. _____in the home does great damage to the immune system of a female.   page 132

Our findings are that MCS/EI is the result of a relationship breakup in the person's life, usually with a close family member. One or more of five life circumstances contribute to this breakdown. These five life circumstances are: (1) verbal abuse (2) emotional abuse (3) physical abuse (4) sexual abuse and (5) drivenness to meet the expectation of a parent. The need to receive love can cause a person to become driven to meet the expectation of a parent.

MCS/EI is an anxiety disease that compromises the immune system to the degree that allergies develop. The only way to get healed of MCS/EI is to break the anxiety syndrome, or pattern, so that the immune system can heal.

3.   When the immune system heals, the peripheral conditions, such as candida, fibromyalgia, hypothyroidism, will no longer exist in the body. These conditions are caused by a _____ _____.   page 133

Trying to heal the bad fruit of fear and stress is not a more excellent way. Solving the root problem IS a more excellent way.

How does an allergist approach the disease? An allergist starts from the outside by having people avoid things like certain foods and environments.

4. God says in His Word that everything he made was not just "good;" He said it was _____ _____.

> And God saw every thing that he had made, and, behold, it was very good. And the evening and the morning were the sixth day.
>
> Genesis 1:31

From an article in *The Dallas Morning News*:

> Hormones in the body released during stress and depression contribute to brittle bones, infections, and even cancer.
>
> The fight or flight reflex was intended to give endurance to escape danger. The reflex is triggered daily in modern life. It keeps a body in a state of hyper-readiness.
>
> When fight or flight hormones such as cortisol remain unregulated in the body for a long time, disease can result. Studies have shown that depressed women with high levels of these hormones have loss of bone density.

5. The root of depression is _____, _____ and _____. page 134

> For where envying and strife is, there is confusion and every evil work. James 3:16

Fear is not just an emotion. The Bible calls fear an evil spirit.

> For God hath not given us the spirit of fear; but of power, and of love, and of a sound mind.
>
> 2 Timothy 1:7

In order for people to be healed of MCS/EI,
they need freedom on two levels:
spiritual and psychological.

Mankind is programmed on two levels: the spirit man and the intellect. Your long-term memory locks the object of your fears into your mind. These fears are your stressors.

MCS/EI Reaction Illustrated

When you are facing your stressor – the forbidden food or smell, or someone says, "The bug man is here," you are programmed to think that it (the forbidden food), or he (the bug man) is the enemy. Instantly there is a hormone generated by the hypothalamus that goes into the bloodstream. The heart and respiratory rates increase, rapidity of breathing begins, and it can go from slow to panic, instantly. A state of anaphylaxis can result. Catatonic realities can result. Death can result.

Hyperventilation results from two things: reduction of oxygen at the upper level of the brain and increase of carbon dioxide levels.

6. Hyperventilation interferes with getting proper fuel to your brain cells. This causes brain _____. The medical diagnosis is often "organic brain syndrome." page 139

Loss of concentration follows and increases fear. With that fear, more hormones are released. Then hyperventilation increases. Catatonic reality and anaphylaxis result until the stressors have passed.

When the stressor is removed, this ends the temporary EI reaction.

The first stage of the General Adaptation Syndrome (GAS) is called the "alarm stage."

7.   After the alarm stage, the _____ _____ begins. page 139

People who do not have an anxiety disorder resume a normal lifestyle when this episode is over. People with anxiety disorders never leave fight or flight. Fear of the "stressor" is always there.

8.   The last stage of the GAS is called the _____ stage when all the peripheral diseases start to develop. You can read about the progression of diseases in *A More Excellent Way*™, 7th Edition, pages 141-148.

How does the body react?

The thyroid gland is first to be affected. Hypothyroidism is often a part of this profile. The liver becomes impaired. The adrenal cortex is behind it. The elimination of H+ ions, water retention and sodium retention occurs. This affects the ionic base, the acidic levels and the alkalinity levels.

Candida comes, bringing pain as well as low self-esteem. Fibromyalgia is the next response of the body. Fibromyalgia is pain that has no organic reason. Hopelessness, despair and more fear result. Fear of doctors and medical treatments intensify the situation even more.

Can it be healed?

Yes, you can break this cycle by:

- Not being afraid
- Not looking at your symptoms
  (They are a lie.)
- Knowing you are not alone in this disease anymore.

If the resistance stage fails to combat the stressor and the body gives up, the disease will push the body to the third and final stage of this fear-anxiety disorder. What happens in the final stage of the General Adaptation Syndrome? The body loses potassium ions, and goes into exhaustion.

This ministry is convinced that MCS/EI is a disease of the broken heart.

How do we approach ministry to people suffering from MCS/EI? First bring them to reconciliation.

- Reconciliation to God
- Reconciliation to themselves
- Reconciliation towards others

There has to be reconciliation in the heart on all three levels. Love is a major factor in being healed.

There is no fear in love; but perfect love casts out fear: because fear hath torment. He that feareth is not made perfect in love. 1 John 4:18

Increased fear means more destruction
to the immune system
and more allergic reactions.

Is fight or flight part of our creation? Yes. But we have an enemy that wants to make fight or flight a permanent way of life. Adrenaline is released in the body during fight or flight, but fight or flight does not eliminate the invisible enemy. The enemy does not go away, but gets progressively stronger in programming us.

The spiritual elements of MCS/EI are:

- Great insecurity, not feeling loved
- Great fear
- Great mistrust

MCS/EI stands on fear and occultism.

Fear is occultism
because it projects into the future
something that is not true
as if it were true.

9. The elements of healing for MCS/EI are: to trust again and be _____. page 142

The Endocrine System

10. The hypothalamus is called the _____ of the endocrine system. It is located in the third ventricle. When the back of your head hurts from tension, this is where you rub your neck. It is the

facilitator for many things, and this is covered more fully later under the limbic system. page 143

11. An EI reaction is a direct result of a combination of hormones being secreted by the _____, and the central nervous system being activated by fear, anxiety and stress. page 143

In order for people to be healed of MCS/EI, the spirit of fear has to be removed from their life.

12. When you are continually geared up to fight a stressor, there are all kinds of things happening inside your body. Science calls it the mind-body connection. We call it the spirit, soul and _____ connection. page 145

Limbic System

The limbic system is the connection between your cerebrum, where your brain is, down through to your hypothalamus. It is the connection between the psyche (thought) and the physio (body).

God is not only interested in your spirit that will go to heaven one day, but also in your day-to-day survival. Psychology teaches that there is a conscious and a collective unconscious part of the soul. The Bible teaches that there is a spirit, a soul and a body.

> And the very God of peace sanctify you wholly; and I pray God your whole spirit and soul and body be preserved blameless unto the coming of our Lord Jesus Christ.
>
> 1 Thessalonians 5:23

The hypothalamus is called the "brain" of the endocrine system, but it is not a brain. It is a gland, which is a facilitator and originator of the following life circumstances: fear, anxiety, stress, tension, panic, panic attacks, phobia, rage, anger and aggression.

> Peace I leave with you, my peace I give unto you: not as the world giveth, give I unto you. Let not your heart be troubled, neither let it be afraid.   John 14:27

13. In Isaiah 9:6, Jesus is called the _____ of Peace.

> *The antidote to fear*
> *is fellowship with the Godhead.*
> *If you are listening to fear,*
> *you are not listening to God.*

The limbic system functions in the emotional aspects of behavior related to survival. When you do not feel loved or secure, or have been victimized, you fight for survival. The limbic system also functions in memory and controls most of the involuntary aspects of the entire nervous system.

General Adaptation Syndrome (GAS)

Homeostasis may be viewed as a specific response by the body to specific stimuli. Its mechanisms "fine tune" the body, and if successful, our environment maintains a uniform chemistry, temperature and pressure. However, if stress is extreme or unusual, the stress triggers a wide-ranging set of bodily changes called General Adaptation Syndrome (GAS).

14. GAS does not maintain a constant internal environment. In fact, it does just the opposite. The purpose of these changes is to gear up the body to meet emergencies, known as _____.

A stressor is anything that causes fear in your life. Reread *A More Excellent Way*™, 7th Edition, page 151 to see the parts of the body that one stressor can affect on a long-term basis.

> *Fear and anxiety are affecting your body*
> *behind the scenes,*
> *and you do not even see it happening.*

Cortisol

Cortisol is a very important hormone in the body in fight or flight. However, the long-term, oversecretion of cortisol destroys your immune system, and according to the medical community, has direct physiological effects on a lot of bodily functions that you can read about on page 152.

> **A merry heart doeth good like a medicine:**
> **but a broken spirit drieth the bones.**
> Proverbs 17:22

As we go into fear and self-rejection,
our body takes on a profile of death
because our thoughts have spiritually murdered us.

When you deny your existence as God sees you,
and you reject yourself in creation,
a spirit of death comes.

Are you rejecting yourself instead of loving yourself?

If so,
you are disagreeing with God
and opening yourself to a spirit of death.

Cortisol directly influences immune responses to antibodies. It inhibits the production of macrophages and helper T cells. Diminished helper T cells cause a decrease in B cells and antibody production. This begins the destruction of the immune system.

When we eliminate the root problem,
the rest of the body will conform to health as God intended.

Cardiovascular System

The cardiovascular system is the target organ system for fear, anxiety and stress.

Angina (Pain)

Angina occurs as three primary types. Angina pectoris is most commonly known. The word in the Greek language literally means "a strangling." This definition includes severe pain in the chest associated with emotional stress and characterized by feelings of suffocation and apprehension. Hyperactivity of the sympathetic nervous system, produced by the hypothalamus in relationship to the mind-body connection, is clearly implicated in the medical journals.

> **Men's hearts failing them for fear...**   Luke 21:26

High Blood Pressure (Hypertension)

This is the result of a narrowing of the blood vessels so that there is a resistance to the flow, thus increasing the pressure because of the backup in the coronary vessels.

Pastor Henry is not opposed to medical science. What he sees is that the Bible only proves medical science and medical science only proves the Bible. He finds no conflict. It is just that the third dimension of our existence, which is the spirit of man, is usually not recognized in the scientific and medical community.

> *It is essential to understand*
> *that man is not just a soul and a body*
> *but is also a spirit.*
> *Problems are spiritual first.*

Heart Arrhythmias

These are disturbances of heart rhythm or other arrhythmic problems. Not only can the heart be stimulated by chemical messengers, but through the involuntary nervous system, it is neurologically sensitive to thought via the mind-body connection.

Because of this neurological reason, the heartbeat can be interrupted. It would be like cutting the electrical current to something off, and then turning it back on.

Mitral Valve Prolapse (Heart Valve Disease)

15. This is similar to arrhythmic problems. The reality of fear, anxiety and stress upstream in the spirit and the soul causes a whole sequence of events to go into motion through the _____-body connection so the electrical connection to the valve is interrupted.

Conditions Coming out of Self-Bitterness, Self-Rejection and Self-Hatred

Coronary Artery Disease

This is the number one cause of heart attacks. It involves blockage so that oxygen is prevented from reaching the heart muscle, and involves hardening of the arteries, which effectively leads to a narrowing of the arteries.

Strokes

16. Strokes result from the _____ of blood vessels which causes the brain tissue to be blood-starved. In some cases there can be a hemorrhage that also interferes with the function by cutting off a part of its blood supply. This is not to be confused with an aneurysm. page 158

The mechanism that produces this inflammation has an autoimmune component in which the white corpuscles are congregating in the heart muscle, and the nonbacterial inflammation is a by-product. This can be quite serious in heart tissue because the heart can quit beating. This profile also includes fear, anxiety and stress.

Have you noticed when you have an autoimmune disease that self-hatred is always part of the profile?

In Matthew 22:39,
the second commandment Jesus gave was,
"Thou shalt love thy neighbor as thyself."

Conditions Coming out of Anger, Rage and Resentment

Aneurysms

Aneurysms involve either the swelling or the rupturing of blood vessels. When there are exploding blood vessels or bulging blood vessels, you will find anger, rage and resentment in that person. This disease is a highly inherited spiritual disease.

> [26]Be ye angry, and sin not: let not the sun go
> down upon your wrath:
> [27]neither give place to the devil.
> Ephesians 4:26-27

Varicose Veins

These are a form of aneurysms and involve a swelling of blood vessel walls.

Hemorrhoids

17. Hemorrhoids are varicose _____.
Anger, rage and resentment is not always externally explosive against others. It can be internalized, but it is still sin. The result is still the same. page 159

Thrombophlebitis (Vein inflammation)

This primarily affects the body's superficial veins, which are easily seen on the surface of the skin, especially in the legs. It is common in people with varicose veins.

Heart Problems — Congenital, Inherited or Injury in Utero

A defect of the heart or major blood vessels can be present at birth. Congenital heart disease is found in 7 out of every 1,000 births. If a child is born with a heart disease, Pastor Henry would consider this to be the inherited genetic curse (iniquity). We minister by simply asking God to do a creative miracle and restore the tissue that has been damaged.

Muscles

Tension Headaches, Muscle Contraction Backache

Fear, anxiety and stress are the spiritual roots of both tension headaches and muscle contraction backaches.

Connective Tissue Disease, Rheumatoid Arthritis

Pastor Henry does not agree with the medical community as to fear, anxiety and stress being the root.

139

A person with rheumatoid arthritis does not want to face themselves, and out of that comes self-hatred, and out of that comes guilt, and out of that comes the conflict that causes the white corpuscles to attack and eat the connective material of the bones. In Unit Eight, it says this includes the joints of the skeleton, the tissues and the cartilage.

Inflammatory Diseases of Connective Tissue

Prostatitis

There are two types of inflammation, which are bacterial and nonbacterial. Bacterial is treated with antibiotics. Nonbacterial inflammation is caused either by an oversecretion of histamine, or by an excess of white corpuscles that localize and cause the inflammation. Prostatitis is a male disease.

Interstitial Cystitis

Interstitial Cystitis is a female disease comparable to prostatitis.

Pulmonary System

Asthma (called Hypersensitivity Reaction)

18. John Hopkins University Research Team confirmed that it has nothing to do with what you breathe. It can be inherited, but it is coming out of deep-rooted fear, anxiety and _____.
    Pastor Henry identified fear of abandonment coupled with insecurity as the specific fear issue.
    page 160

Hay Fever

19. This is a hypersensitivity reaction. This is antigen-antibody relative to a compromised _____ system, and is a fear, anxiety and stress disorder. page 161

Immune System

Immunosuppression or Deficiency

As you continue to attack yourself spiritually with self-rejection, self-hatred and self-bitterness, the body finally agrees and the white corpuscles start to attack your body.

Autoimmune Diseases

20. These are primarily self-hatred diseases with a fear, anxiety, stress rider attached to them. The body attacks the body because the person is attacking himself or herself spiritually in three "self" conflicts which are self-rejection, self-hatred and self-bitterness, coupled with guilt. The _____ spirit also produces feelings of not being loved and not being accepted. As the person continues to attack himself or herself spiritually, the body finally agrees and the white corpuscles are invisibly redirected to attack living tissue while ignoring the true enemy, which is bacteria and viruses. page 161

Some people with autoimmune diseases
said that they were told
that it was caused by self-hatred,
but they couldn't see it.

Stop and take a good long look.

Are you mad at your body
because it is not performing
the way you want it to?

How do you expect your body
to work for you if you hate it?

Some of the autoimmune diseases include lupus, diabetes, rheumatoid arthritis, MS and Crohn's disease, which is similar to ulcerative colitis, as it can ulcerate because of the attack of the white corpuscles on the lining of the colon.

Gastrointestinal System

Ulcers

21. With ulcers, the dendrites are flaring in the lining of the _____. People who have ulcers also have a compromised immune system, and when they do, they do not have the firepower to defeat bacteria. Pastor Henry thinks that fear, anxiety and stress came first, and the bacteria showed up after the immune system was compromised. page 162

Irritable Bowel Syndrome (IBS)

The dendrites are flaring in the lining of the colon. This is similar to what's happening in the lining of the stomach that produces ulcers.

Diarrhea

22. Diarrhea can be caused by continual irritation in conjunction with the _____ malfunctioning as part of the profile of the GAS of fear, anxiety and stress. page 162

Constipation

Constipation has the same spiritual root as diarrhea.

Nausea and Vomiting

This can be caused by a nervous stomach, or as a result of fear, anxiety and stress, or excessive gastric activity in conjunction with the central nervous system.

Ulcerative Colitis

23. The lining of the colon is irritated by excessive flaring of the _____ to the degree that the lining ulcerates and bleeds. page 162

Malabsorption (Leaky Gut)

The food being digested and the nutrients from it never reach the cellular level through the bloodstream. A high percentage of the digested food, including expensive health food and supplements, just passes on through, resulting in various stages of malnutrition.

Genitourinary System

Diuresis

This is excessive bladder elimination. Many times incontinence may also be found in fear, anxiety and stress disorders.

Impotence

Statistics indicate that as many as 40 percent of all men in America have impotence. The spiritual roots are fear, anxiety and stress coming out of self-rejection and lack of self-esteem.

Frigidity

24. This is a female disorder. As a female's _____ system has been compromised, many times sexual identity and uncleanness in it can be implicated. page 163

Skin

Eczema

This involves itching, redness, inflammation and occasionally pustules. There could also be implications of excessive histamine secretion and excessive autoimmune activity. This is clearly identified in Deuteronomy 28 as a curse resulting from disobedience to God and His Word.

Neurodermatitis

This is a chronic inflammation of the skin. It may have a strong psychogenic component that is a very definite spiritual root involving anxiety, mental tension and emotional disturbances. It is definitely a result of the mind-body connection. Females deal with this more than males.

Acne

This disorder is usually on the face, neck, back and shoulders. Medical research has identified adolescent acne as fear, anxiety and stress that is a result of peer pressure. Kids are afraid of other kids. This triggers increased histamine secretion behind the skin and also increases the secretion of oil in the epidermis.

Endocrine System

Diabetes Mellitus

25. The medical community puts this in the fear, anxiety and stress category. Pastor Henry says that fear, anxiety and stress is a rider attached to the disease, but that it is an autoimmune disease. The spiritual roots are self-hatred and self-rejection coupled with guilt, but the bigger root cause that allows these to come is the _____ spirit. page 164

Amenorrhea

This is an interruption or stoppage of the menstrual cycle in females. The medical community defines the root as emotional stress or depression. In this ministry, many women, after dealing with fear, anxiety and stress, have resumed their menstrual cycles as a part of their healing, even after stoppage for many years.

Central Nervous System

Fatigue and Lethargy

This is found under the third stage of the General Adaptation Syndrome and is called exhaustion. Many medical manuals attribute it to fear, anxiety and stress.

26. Exhaustion, fatigue and lethargy are by-products of the root problem of hypoglycemia, which is a reduction in glucose levels. It is primarily a fear, anxiety and stress disorder with an _____ rider attached to it coming out of fear, self-hatred and guilt. page 165

Type A Behavior

27. This involves drivenness, performance and perfectionism. A root can include fear of poverty, or the need to succeed in order to be _____ or accepted. Another root is the expectation put on someone by a parent or spouse. page 165

Do you see yourself in this?
Maybe you do not consider yourself a driven person,
but just think about times when you really pushed
to get something right in order to please someone.

Are you a people-pleaser?
Are you doing it to gain love?
Do you have "fear of man?"

Overeating

28. Overeating is a false comforter. Four powerful forces drive this, producing long-term fear, anxiety and stress. They are fear of rejection,

fear of man, fear of failure and fear of
_____. page 165

A person who is driven burns large amounts of fuel supply which produces a chemical need for nutrition replacement beyond the normal.

Depression

29. This is a result of chemical imbalance in the body. It is produced by conflict at the spirit or _____ level in which the limbic system responds to this stress. Depression is a result of the chemical imbalance produced by the body in response. page 165

Insomnia

The hypothalamus gland regulates sleep, so if this gland senses conflict or fear, anxiety and stress, it responds and interferes with the peace of this person.

Fear, Anxiety and Stress Disorders

First John 4:18 is the foundational scripture for the healing of many fear, anxiety and stress disorders including MCS/EI. There are four parts of this verse, and each must be individually read, recognized and digested to apply them to our lives.

30. Note: "There is no fear in _____..." If you are not loved perfectly, then fear comes. That is the fear that causes these diseases. Part two says "...perfect love casteth out fear..." page 167

All spiritually rooted diseases that are caused by fear involve a breach in relationship. The three areas of separation are separation from God, separation from yourself and separation from others.

Most people misunderstand the term "to fear the LORD." There are fourteen different Hebrew words and seven different Greek words translated into English as "fear." When referring to "fear of God," it has to do with reverential respect because we honor Him for who He is.

31. Part three of 1 John 4:18 says "...because fear hath _____..." That is what causes many mental and psychological diseases, either through the inherited component of genetics or the inherited familiar spirits (iniquity) that come to produce it. Most of the things that happen in our head occur because we are afraid. page 168

32. Part four says, "...He that feareth is not made perfect in love." You have fear because you have a breach somewhere in your relationships at some level. This allowed the _____, unclean spirit to attach itself to you. page 168

If you are not able to give and receive love, then you have fear.

Anti-anxiety and antidepressant drugs are not the answer for fear. These are neurological blockers and calming agents with extremely dangerous side effects. They are a form of disease management, and are a poor substitute for the peace of God.

We trust you have gained insight into the spiritual roots of many diseases that are coming out of fear, anxiety and stress. There is *a more excellent way!*

Answers to Unit Seven

1. broken spirit
2. strife
3. root problem
4. very good
5. fear, stress and anxiety
6. fog
7. resistance stage
8. exhaustion
9. vulnerable
10. brain
11. hypothalamus
12. body
13. Prince
14. stressors
15. mind
16. clogging
17. veins
18. stress
19. immune
20. unloving
21. stomach
22. liver
23. dendrites
24. value

25. unloving

26. autoimmune

27. loved

28. abandonment

29. soul

30. love

31. torment

32. unloving

Study Unit Eight:
Specific Diseases

See *A More Excellent Way*™, 7th Edition, pages 171–252*

The following insights about diseases are hypotheses coming from case histories. They are listed in alphabetical order.

If you are taking prescription drugs,
do not come off of your medication
without the supervision of a doctor.

Acne

Skin: page 214
Spiritual Insight: What they have discovered, for the most part, is that adolescent acne is rooted in anxiety and fear coming out of peer pressure. Simple acne is coming out of fear of man. It is fear of rejection and fear of man.

Acne (Cystic)

See Ovarian Cysts

Addictions

Addictive Personality: page 243
Spiritual Insight: All addictions are rooted in the need to be loved. In dealing with addictions, dopamine is very important to pay attention to because it is the pleasure neurotransmitter of the human body.

Addictive Personality:

page 248

---

* Page numbers refer to *A More Excellent Way*™

Description: In anorexia the person refuses to eat. In bulimia people eat, but purge themselves of the food just eaten. Bulimia also includes excessive eating in exchange for the void of not feeling loved.

Spiritual Insight: The roots are the same: self-hatred, self-rejection and guilt, which effectively cause the serotonin levels to become deficient. Again, when you have lowered serotonin levels, the spiritual and emotional feelings of unloveliness are now reinforced by the chemical deficiency.

> *Have you ever wondered why some people*
> *can drink and are not alcoholics,*
> *and others drink and are alcoholics?*

Alcoholism

Addictive Personality: page 244

Spiritual Insight: Alcoholism runs in families because there is a curse in those families that produces it. There is also a genetic component to consider. The success with alcoholism comes first of all from the Lord delivering the person, in conjunction with him or her just having had enough. There has to come a time in the person's life where he or she makes a quality decision to just say "NO."

Allergies

page 232

Description: An allergy is a hypersensitive reaction to any antigen (any substance that produces a reaction).

Spiritual Insight: long-term fear, anxiety and stress can destroy your immune system, and when that happens you have antigen to antibody. That is exactly what an allergy is, a hypersensitive reaction.

Your body is not allergic to anything.
God created you to be compatible
with everything that you are exposed to.
What did the devil do to you,
through a sequence of events,
that brought fear, anxiety and stress
to destroy your immune system?

Alzheimer's Disease

page 210

Description: According to recent research, it seems to involve a proliferation of white corpuscles that are congregating at critical nerve junctions in the brain.

Spiritual Insight: Whenever white corpuscles are attacking the body and not doing what God created them to do there are various degrees of self-hatred and guilt.

Angina Pectoris

Cell Membrane Rigidity: page 193

Description: Angina is a cell membrane rigidity disease that involves the hardening and stiffening and narrowing of blood vessels and produces reduced coronary circulation.

Spiritual Insight: Stress and anxiety is a common cause. It produces a constriction of vessel walls. Also implicated is strenuous exercise or a heavy meal. Apprehension and dread increases the problem.

> Men's hearts failing them for fear, and for looking after those things which are coming on the earth: for the powers of heaven shall be shaken.   Luke 21:26

Arthritis (Involving Inflammation of the Joints)

page 190

Description: Simple arthritis is the inflammation of a joint usually accompanied by pain, swelling and frequently changes in structure.

Spiritual Insight: The spiritual root for simple arthritis involves bitterness against others.

Asthma

Cell Membrane Rigidity: page 192

Description: There is stiffening of the cell walls of the alveoli. This causes an entrapment of carbon dioxide and an exclusion of oxygen. Thus you have breathing problems.

Spiritual Insight: Asthma is a fear-anxiety manifestation. It can be inherited. We have observed from medical journals that the hypothalamus gland, when it senses fear and anxiety, causes a hormone called ACTH to be secreted. This hormone goes into the bloodstream and docks at a receptor cell in the alveoli. This produces the stiffening. Fear of abandonment and the resulting insecurities is the key issue behind asthma.

Attention Deficit Disorder

page 194

Description: There are three types: a combined attention deficit type, an inattentive type and hyperactive impulsive type. The high range is hyperactivity. ADD is a neurological interruption that seems to run in family trees. Also see Merck Manual, 17th Edition, page 2255.

Spiritual Insight: ADD is coming out of a dumb and deaf spirit. There is a double mindedness that comes, and this is an inherited family curse. The prime root of the confusion is gender disorientation because of an inversion of godly order in the home. The home is ruled by matriarchal control rather than patriarchal authority as God intended. There are also various standpoints of rebellion as part of this profile. Historic family rebellion exists in families that have been involved in occultism and false religions. Historically, it is an interrupter of the thoughts. It interferes with self-esteem. It involves much self-rejection, self-hatred and guilt.

> *When the male does not rule the home in love,*
> *as a spiritual covering,*
> *the female has no choice but to take the reins.*
> *The minute she does,*
> *Satan's entire kingdom comes to help her.*
> *She was never designed to rule the home;*
> *she was designed to follow a godly patriarch.*

[3]But I would have you know, that the head of every man is Christ; and the head of the woman *is* the man; and the head of Christ *is* God.

1 Corinthians 11:3

Autism

page 209

Description: Recent medical research indicates that an imbalance in a particular neurotransmitter secretion is implicated.

Spiritual Insight: It is possible that autism is a result of rejection. The other components of autism involve rebellion and anger.

Bipolar Disorder

See Manic Depression

Breast Cancer

page 183

Spiritual Insight: Breast Cancer is coming out of the sins of conflict and bitterness between the female and either her mother or her sisters or mother-in-law.

Cysts or tumors that appear in the left breast tissue seem to follow unresolved bitterness and conflict between that female and another female blood relative, such as mother, sister, aunt, grandmother.

Cysts or tumors that appear in the right breast tissue seem to follow unresolved bitterness and conflict between that female and another female (non-blood relative), such as a mother-in-law or a person in the workplace or a person in the church.

The target cells in females are in the breast tissue because the breasts are the nurturing aspect of a female.

Editor's Note: Ten percent of all breast cancer is caused by mammograms.

Breast Cysts

See Ovarian Cysts

Bulimia

See Anorexia and Bulimia

Cell Membrane Rigidity
versus
Cell Membrane Permeability

In normal tissue, when you have cell membrane permeability, it means that through osmosis, material in the bloodstream necessary for the cell enters through the semi-permeable membrane of the cell, and the waste by-product is exchanged. When you have cell membrane rigidity, you have stiffening of the cell membrane, and osmosis is hindered.

Cholesterol

page 211

Spiritual Insight: High cholesterol is directly related to people who are very angry with themselves. There is a high degree of self-deprecation; they're against themselves, and they always put themselves down.

CFIDS

See CFS

CFS or CFIDS
(Chronic Fatigue Syndrome, Chronic Fatigue Immune Dysfunction Syndrome)

page 235

Description: CFS is characterized by exhaustion and involves a diagnosis of hypoglycemia, low blood sugar. **Spiritual Insight**: Hypoglycemia has an autoimmune component. Someone with an autoimmune disease, without exception, has degrees of lack of self-esteem and guilt. CFS is a very major fear-anxiety disorder and is the result of drivenness to meet the expectation of a parent in order to receive love. The love is usually sought from a mother, but not always.

157

*The word "syndrome" basically means
the medical profession does not know
what causes the disease.
When you hear the words:
"incurable"
"etiology unknown"
or "syndrome,"
you usually have
a spiritually rooted disease.*

Chronic Fatigue Immune Dysfunction Syndrome

See CFS

Chronic Fatigue Syndrome

See CFS

Colic

page 238

Description: Colic is a neurological manifestation in the child that is a direct result of a spirit of fear coming in at conception, in utero or at birth.

Spiritual Insight: Colic can be from an inherited spirit of fear. Many times it is inherited from the mother.

Colon Cancer

Cancer: page 181

Spiritual Insight: It is deeply rooted in bitterness and slander with the tongue. It can be inherited.

**When you speak evil against someone, it is a curse.
What you speak against another returns to you.**

Death and life *are* in the power of the tongue:
and they that love it shall eat the fruit thereof.
Proverbs 18:21

Crohn's Disease

The Immune System: page 174

Description: The white corpuscles start attacking the lining of the colon causing ulceration and extreme bleeding. Although primarily in the colon, it can appear in the ileum, the esophagus and at any point of the gastrointestinal tract in advanced cases of spreading.

Spiritual Insight: As we attack ourselves spiritually, the body eventually agrees and starts attacking itself in destruction. The roots are extreme self-rejection and guilt. It can come out of massive rejection, abandonment, lack of self-esteem or drivenness to meet the expectation of another. It involves conflict, hopelessness, codependency and false burden bearing.

Degenerative Disc Disease

page 223

Description: Anything dealing with the disc, apart from accidents and injury, that is degenerative in nature.

Spiritual Insight: Inherited or degenerative disc disease is usually tied to an addictive personality involving drugs, both legal and illegal. Somewhere in your family line there may be someone who was a drug runner or put drugs or alcohol to someone else's lips to make them drunk or your own usage of such.

Have you noticed that many people coming out of the "Hippie" days have back problems?

> [15]Woe unto him that giveth his neighbour drink, that puttest thy bottle to *him,* and makest *him* drunken also, that thou mayest look on their nakedness!

> [16]Thou art filled with shame for glory: drink thou also, and let thy foreskin be uncovered: the cup of the LORD's right hand shall be turned unto thee, and shameful spewing *shall be* on thy glory.
> Habakkuk 2:15-16

Diabetes

See Hyperglycemia

Diabetes 1

Autoimmune Disease: page 176

Description: Diabetes 1 is an autoimmune disease. It is a disorder of the endocrine system where the white corpuscles attack the pancreas affecting its ability to produce or utilize insulin.

Spiritual Insight: The root is extreme rejection coupled with guilt. There is direct rejection by a father, a husband or a man in general resulting in a broken heart. It can also come from an inherited unloving spirit. It can be inherited from both a genetic and spiritual standpoint.

Dissociative Identity Disorder
(formerly Multiple Personality Disorder)

page 228

Spiritual Insight: Biblically there seems to be evidence that DID is actually the kingdom called Legion. "We are many" is called Legion. In Mark 5 when Legion was removed, the person was in his right mind.

> And he asked him, What is thy name? And he answered, saying, My name is Legion: for we are many.
> Mark 5:9

Endometriosis

page 219

Spiritual Insight: Possibly rooted in self-rejection and self-hatred.

Epilepsy

page 200

Description: Seizure disorders.

Spiritual Insight: The dumb and deaf spirit and a spirit of epilepsy are found in epilepsy and need to be cast out.

Psychologists have been able to document
that many of our personality characteristics
including rage, anger,
predisposition to mental disorders
and certain diseases,
can be found in humans without any genetic component,
but it can still be inherited.
How is that possible?
What is the origin of these thoughts?

Fibromyalgia

page 216

Description: Fibromyalgia is an appropriate term for pain where inflammation is absent.

Spiritual Insight: Fibromyalgia, for the most part, is rooted in fear, anxiety, stress, drivenness and perfectionism. It can be found in females who do not feel covered, protected and nurtured.

Most female disorders are the result
of a lack of nurturing and protection (covering) by a male.
The female is then saddled with the problems of life
without any help, emotionally or spiritually.
The cause is anxiety, stress and fear
coming upon a woman under those circumstances
because she was not made to be the stronger vessel.
The Bible says, she has been created
to be the weaker vessel.

> Likewise, ye husbands, dwell with *them*
> according to knowledge, giving honour unto the
> wife, as unto the weaker vessel, and as being
> heirs together of the grace of life; that your
> prayers be not hindered.   1 Peter 3:7

It does not mean that she's weak upstairs.
It does not mean that she's weak before God.
It means that in the God-ordained order of things,
she is designed to respond and be a helpmeet to her husband.

Flu

page 238

Spiritual Insight: There is no spiritual root behind the
flu necessarily. "Often infirmities" are things that are
common to man that are in the earth because of
bacterium and other aspects of Adam's fall. They do
not necessarily have a spiritual root as such, but are a
part of the fall of man.

> Many *are* the afflictions of the righteous: but
> the LORD delivereth him out of them all.
>   Psalm 34:19

Editor's note: An uncompromised immune system will combat infirmities.

Graves' Disease

See Hyperthyroidism

Hashimoto's Disease

See Hypothyroidism

Herpes

Virus: page 181
Description: Herpes is a virus.
Spiritual Insight: Herpes seems to go into remission, but under stress it erupts.

God created our immune system to fight off invaders. If our immune system does not fight off an infirmity, then is there a spiritual reason that caused our immune system to be compromised?

High Blood Pressure

See Hypertension

Hives

See Shingles and Hives

Hodgkin's Disease and Leukemia

page 186
Spiritual Insight: Hodgkin's disease and leukemia, many times, are caused by deep-rooted bitterness coming from unresolved rejection by a father, abandonment by a father — either literally or emotionally.

Hyperglycemia (Diabetes)

page 240
Description: It involves high blood sugar and there is much evidence of an autoimmune component attached to it. It is an autoimmune disease with an anxiety rider.

Spiritual Insight: Autoimmune diseases are indicative of self-hatred and guilt, but there is also a root of fear, stress and anxiety.

Hypertension (High Blood Pressure)

Cell Membrane Rigidity: page 193

Description: Cell membrane rigidity which produces a vasoconstriction of blood vessels, coupled with an increase of cardiac output which increases the blood pressure.

Spiritual Insight: It is caused by fear and anxiety.

> *What were the open doors in a person's life,*
> *either inherited or personal,*
> *that allowed a spirit of fear to come in*
> *and control him or her?*

For God hath not given us the spirit of fear;
but of power, and of love, and of a sound mind.
2 Timothy 1:7

Editor's note: Fear of tomorrow is the specific root of hypertension.

Hyperthyroidism (Graves' Disease)

page 241

Description: An oversecretion of thyroxin. It can produce goiters and swelling of the eyes and palpitations and tremors.

Spiritual Insight: It is primarily an anxiety disorder that also involves self-hatred, self-rejection and guilt. The primary triggering point for Graves' can be the result of emotional shock or a prolonged period of anxiety.

Hypoglycemia (Low Blood Sugar)

page 240

Description: Hypoglycemia is low blood sugar.

Spiritual Insight: It is rooted in anxiety and fear coupled with self-hatred and self-rejection coupled with guilt. Also lack of identity, insecurity and performance orientation may also be implicated.

Hypothyroidism (Hashimoto's Disease)

page 241

Description: The manifestation of lowered levels of thyroxin being secreted by the thyroid. It is an anxiety disorder with an autoimmune component.

Spiritual Insight: Beginning from fear, anxiety and stress, the advanced stage has self-hatred, self-rejection and guilt as the major root with fear, anxiety and stress becoming a rider component.

Immune System

God created your immune system to maintain your body and fight off invaders. In all autoimmune diseases the immune system begins to destroy your body.

Interstitial Cystitis

Nonbacterial Inflammation: page 190

Description: Interstitial cystitis is a swelling and inflammation of the bladder tissue of females.

Spiritual Insight: Its root is a combination of anxiety, fear, guilt and self-hatred.

Irritable Bowel Syndrome

page 238

Description: Irritable bowel syndrome (IBS) is caused by the misfiring of nerve dendrites in the lining of the intestine.

Spiritual Insight: IBS is coming directly out of anxiety, fear and insecurities.

Leukemia

See Hodgkin's Disease and Leukemia

Liver Cancer

Cancer: page 183

Spiritual Insight: Liver cancer sometimes can be connected to sexual sin.

Is it possible that there is a warning from the Word of God concerning the fruit of being addicted to pornographic material?

> [21]With her much fair speech she caused him to yield, with the flattering of her lips she forced him.
> [22]He goeth after her straightway, as an ox goeth to the slaughter, or as a fool to the correction of the stocks;
> [23]Till a dart strike through his liver; as a bird hasteth to the snare, and knoweth not that it *is* for his life.   Proverbs 7:21-23

Low Blood Sugar

See Hypoglycemia

Lupus

Autoimmune Disease: page 177

Description: Lupus is an autoimmune disease in which the white corpuscles attack the connective tissue of the organs.

Spiritual Insight: Lupus is rooted in extreme self-hatred, self-conflict and includes guilt. Performance also may be implicated.

Manic Depression (Bipolar Disorder)

Genetically Inherited Disease: page 172

Description: A genetic defect disease in which a recessive gene is passed down through the mother. This defect produces a reduction in the secretion of serotonin.

Spiritual Insight: God can deliver a person from the depression and anxiety, and the secretion of serotonin will come back into balance. Drugs which are serotonin enhancers can interfere in dealing with root problems because they mask the real issues.

Editor's Note: If you are taking prescription drugs, do not come off of your medication without the supervision of a doctor.

If it were God's will that you be artificially maintained, why didn't He set in motion artificial maintenance programs for His people?

Masturbation

Addictive Personality: page 244

Spiritual Insight: Masturbation usually begins in childhood, not necessarily because of lust, but coming out of families that are full of strife. A child growing up in an atmosphere full of tension and strife will get temporary relief from masturbating, because an orgasm releases dopamine. But what comes in behind it are the feelings of uncleanness and guilt. Masturbation and cocaine are very similar in their spiritual implications — a release and fulfillment, then guilt and condemnation. Your enemy certainly knows how to work you over!

Migraines

page 229

Description: A migraine is a type of headache pain known as psychogenic pain. Psychogenic means that it is not caused by any known organic reason. It comes and it goes and it is incredibly painful. It brings with it nausea, flashing lights and a complete shutting down of one's ability to cope with life.

Spiritual Insight: Migraines are triggered in people who have conflict with themselves about the conflict in their life or conflict with others. It is rooted in guilt. All migraines are rooted in guilt. Out of guilt comes fear, and it is always in that order.

Mitral Valve Prolapse

page 234

Description: The mitral valve in the heart does not open and shut correctly. This allows blood to flow backward into the atrium causing the heart to work harder.

Spiritual Insight: The root is fear and anxiety.

Multiple Personality Disorder

See Dissociative Identity Disorder

Multiple Sclerosis

page 177

Description: Multiple sclerosis occurs when the white corpuscles attack the myelin sheath, which is the coating of the nerve. The nerve is also damaged. It is the nerve that allows muscles to work.

Spiritual Insight: MS is rooted in deep, deep self-hatred and guilt, and is similar to diabetes in that it involves a father's rejection.

The father is responsible
for the spiritual welfare of the family.
The father, not the mother, is responsible
for the daughter's value system and her self-esteem.

Nutrition

page 249

Spiritual Insight: You need to eat meals three times a day. It is the morning meal that sets metabolism into motion for the rest of the day and burns the calories. Eat something nutritious in the morning and drink plenty of water throughout the day.

Any teaching on nutrition is not going to work if you are negating what nutrition represents by yielding to fear, anxiety and stress. This will cancel the benefits by producing diseases.

Whatever God has created is for you in moderation, without guilt and without self-rejection. You belong here just the way you are. There are ways to lose weight that do not have to be rooted in fear and self-hatred. You can come before God and manage your lifestyle regarding food; and in ministry, deal with unloving spirits, self-hatred, guilt and lack of self-esteem. You can come to a place where you will be comfortable with your body.

Osteoarthritis

Arthritis: page 190

Description: Osteoarthritis is progressive cartilage degeneration in joints and vertebrae and usually does not involve inflammation.

Spiritual Insight: Osteoarthritis is the result of self-bitterness and not forgiving oneself. It is holding a record of wrongs against yourself and also can involve an element of guilt.

When you have bitterness against yourself,
it involves degeneration,
but when you have bitterness against others,
it involves swelling and inflammation.

Osteoporosis

page 220

Spiritual Insight: The healing and prevention of osteoporosis begins in eliminating envy and jealousy from your life.

A sound heart *is* the life of the flesh: but envy the rottenness of the bones.   Proverbs 14:30

Ovarian Cancer

Cancer: page 186

Spiritual Insight: Ovarian cancer comes out of a woman's hatred for herself and her sexuality. Unclean and unloving spirits accuse her about the cleanness of her sexuality and can lead her into self-bitterness and self-loathing concerning her own sexuality.

Ovarian Cysts — Breast Cysts — Cystic Acne

Skin: page 215

Spiritual Insight: These conditions are coming out of the breakup of the relationship between the girl and her mother. Unresolved issues involve a great breach, and there is no fellowship. It carries right down into the reproductive area. It is involved even to the degree that the girl may question her own femininity or the female part of her creation. Many times there is great bitterness, anger and great resentment toward the mother.

Panic Attacks

page 239

Description: A panic attack is an aggressive stage of a fear and anxiety disorder.

Spiritual Insight: It is caused by the spirit of fear.

Paranoid Schizophrenia

page 203

Description: A non-genetic disease of the mind or the soul, which can be inherited. It is the result of a malfunctioning of at least two of the neurotransmitters in the body. It is the result of an oversecretion of norepinephrine and an oversecretion of dopamine.

Spiritual Insight: If you do not want to be vulnerable and transparent, you either withdraw or you create a fabricated personality. Paranoid schizophrenia comes out of fear and rejection, tragedies of your life and victimization. It involves fear of man, fear of rejection, fear of failure, fear of abandonment and unloveliness, guilt, rejection and self-hatred.

*If all of your defense mechanisms were stripped away,
who would you be?
Who has God said you are?
Whose voice are you going to listen to?*

> And Elijah came unto all the people, and
> said, How long halt ye between two opinions? if
> the LORD *be* God, follow him: but if Baal, *then*
> follow him. And the people answered him not a
> word. 1 Kings 18:21

Parasites

page 238

Spiritual Insight: Parasites usually get a long-term foothold because of a compromised immune system. You can have a compromised immune system because of fear, anxiety and stress.

Parkinson's Disease

page 209

Description: Current research is pointing to a deficiency of dopamine as the cause.

Spiritual Insight: Parkinson's is rooted in unresolved rejection, massive amounts of abandonment, rejection and hope deferred.

Phobias

page 240

Description: Phobias are different than panic attacks because phobias are associative and panic can come out of nowhere.

Spiritual Insight: It is caused by the spirit of fear.

The battle is won or lost in the mind.

PMS

See Premenstrual Syndrome

Premenstrual Syndrome (PMS)

page 215

Description: PMS comes from a tightening of the muscles of the uterus and uterine walls, producing pressure, pain, distress and discomfort.

Spiritual Insight: Part of it is tied to fear of pain. Complicating the syndrome also can be feelings of uncleanness around a person's sexuality because of a stigma attached to the monthly cycle. Most people we have seen that have PMS are females who are bound with introspection and stress.

Prostate Cancer

Cancer: page 187

Spiritual Insight: Prostate cancer comes out of anger, guilt, self-hatred and self-bitterness.

All cancer that has a spiritual root involves holding some type of bitterness against yourself or someone else.

[14]We know that we have passed from death unto life, because we love the brethren. He that loveth not *his* brother abideth in death. [15]Whosoever hateth his brother is a murderer: and ye know that no murderer hath eternal life abiding in him. 1 John 3:14-15

Prostatitis

Nonbacterial Inflammation: page 191

Description: Prostatitis is a disease that involves nonbacterial inflammation in males. It involves two dimensions, as does interstitial cystitis, and those are excessive secretion of histamine and a proliferation of white corpuscles on location.

Spiritual Insight: The spiritual root is fear and anxiety, which causes excessive histamine secretion. Self-rejection and self-hatred, coupled with some guilt produces the proliferation of white corpuscles.

Psoriasis

Autoimmune, Skin: page 214

Description: Psoriasis is an autoimmune disorder in which the white corpuscles are congregating on the skin, creating the scaling, the flaking, the redness and the hardness.

Spiritual Insight: Psoriasis is rooted in self-hatred, lack of self-esteem and conflict with identity.

Reflux

page 234

Description: There is a sphincter muscle at the top of your stomach (lower end of your esophagus) and when it does not stay closed, you reflux stomach acid up into the esophagus. This action creates heartburn and even esophageal ulcers.

Spiritual Insight: The root is fear and anxiety.

Rheumatoid Arthritis

Autoimmune Disease: page 178

Description: This is an autoimmune disease where the white corpuscles attack the joints of the skeleton, the tissues, the cartilage and the connective tissue of the skeleton.

Spiritual Insight: As the person attacks himself in self-hatred, so the body conforms to that spiritual dynamic and attacks itself in return. Then a spirit of infirmity comes. The only way to be healed from rheumatoid arthritis and other autoimmune diseases is to accept yourself once and for all.

If God, who is greater than you,
created you, saved you and accepted you,
then why wouldn't you accept yourself?

I will praise thee; for I am fearfully and
wonderfully made: Psalm 139:14

Rosacea

Skin: page 214

Description: Rosacea is a chronic disease of the skin of the face.

Spiritual Insight: Rosacea has more of an autoimmune component to it, rather than anxiety, which involves self-hatred.

Sciatica

page 221

Description: An inflammation of the sciatic nerve that accounts for 50 percent of lower back pain in most people. Medical observation indicates the left side is most usually affected, but it is occasionally the right side.

Spiritual Insight: An evil spirit of sciatica needs to be cast out. (Matthew 10:1 and Luke 10:17-20)

Scoliosis

page 220

Description: Proprioception malfunction is involved. There is a neurological misfiring. One muscle stiffens, and one remains normal, and it gradually causes a curvature of the spine.

Spiritual Insight: Scoliosis, like epilepsy, is the presence and the fruit of an evil spirit. You will not get scoliosis healed, unless you cast out an evil spirit.

Shingles and Hives

Skin: page 212

Description: An acute central nervous system infection involving primarily the dorsal root ganglia and characterized by the vesicular eruption with neuralgic pain in the cutaneous areas, supplied by peripheral sensory nerves arising in the affected root ganglia. Etiology incidents in pathology: herpes zoster is caused by the varicella zoster virus, the same virus that causes chicken pox, and may be activated as local lesions involving the posterior root ganglia by systemic disease.

Spiritual Insight: Shingles is an anxiety and fear disease coupled with an autoimmune component involving self-rejection. Many latent viruses are often released in conjunction with fear. Even though there is a virus implicated in the profile, it is considered an anxiety disorder.

Sinus Infections

page 224

Description: Sinusitis involves the oversecretion of histamine.

Spiritual Insight: The root behind sinus infection and sinusitis is fear and anxiety.

Sjögren's Syndrome

page 239

Description: It is a chronic systemic inflammatory disorder of unknown etiology, characterized by dryness of the mouth, eyes and other mucus membranes.

Spiritual Insight: Since there is an autoimmune component, there would be spiritual roots of extreme self-rejection and self-hatred.

Skin

page 212

When you have an oversecretion of histamine in your body, whether it involves your skin, sinus or an internal organ or tissues, you have swelling. When you have swelling, you have pressure on your nervous system and you have pain, discomfort and irritation. The spiritual root behind this is fear, anxiety and stress over some issue in your life.

Skin Cancer

Cancer: page 183

Spiritual Insight: The evidence seems to involve taking care of the temple (our body) and keeping the skin covered properly to protect it from ultraviolet rays.

Sleep Disorders

page 224

Description: Sleep disorders can be caused by the hypothalamus responding to your spiritual and emotional state.

Spiritual Insight: Certain sleep disorders can be from several sources: fear and anxiety, torment from victimization, or you have not guarded your heart and you have opened up yourself to spirits of fear by the things you watch. If you are not worried about tomorrow, you will sleep tonight. If you are worried about tomorrow, you will not sleep tonight.

So what if you lose everything tomorrow?
The Bible says,
He that would try to save his life
shall lose it,
and he that would lose his life
will save it (Matthew 16:25).

...yea, thou shalt lie down, and thy sleep shall be sweet.   Proverbs 3:24

Thou shalt not be afraid for the terror by night...   Psalm 91:5

Spondylolysis

page 223

Description: Spondylolysis is progressive degeneration of the vertebrae of the spine.

Spiritual Insight: It is rooted in self-hatred.

Toxic Retention

Cell Membrane Rigidity: page 193

Description: When you have cell membrane rigidity, the body will retain various toxins at the cellular level and will not cleanse itself properly because the process of osmosis is hindered.

Spiritual Insight: The spiritual root of the toxic retention is fear and anxiety.

God created your body to cleanse itself of impurities.

...and if they drink any deadly thing, it shall not hurt them...   Mark 16:18

Ulcerative Colitis

pages 174-175

Description: The dendrites flare in the lining of the colon involving irritation, inflammation and ulceration and cause hemorrhaging.

Spiritual Insight: Ulcerative Colitis is an anxiety disorder, not an autoimmune disease. The only way to be healed is to deal with the extreme fear, stress, anxiety and dread that is behind it.

Uterine Cancer

Cancer: page 186

Spiritual Insight: Uterine cancer possibly may be caused by promiscuity and uncleanness; however, behind the promiscuity and the uncleanness is the need to be loved, and that is another issue.

Viruses

Spiritual Insight: A virus does not have its origin with its own life. It is a mutation of the genetic material of an already existing life form. Viruses are difficult to destroy, and seem to have an intelligence behind them because they can mutate, change, hide and even go dormant for years. It is very possible that viruses are spirits of infirmity.

Weight

Addictive Personality: page 246

Spiritual Insight: There is both a genetic and a spiritual component to weight problems. The rate of your metabolism can be determined by how you think about yourself. When you do not feel good about yourself, you go into insecurity. When you are insecure, you start "sucking your thumb." The mouth is a contact place for love and security.

In Conclusion

As the bird by wandering, as the swallow by
flying, so the curse causeless shall not come.

Proverbs 26:2

What can you do
when you do not get well after prayer?
Will you choose the good,
or will you choose evil?
Will you take responsibility,
or will you go into rebellion?
Will you repent?

The bottom line, whether we like it or not,
is submission to the living God,
out of our free will,
because we want to and because we love Him.

He loves us.
He tells us so over and over in His Word.

But when we step
outside the parameters of the covenant,
outside the holiness of God,
then God gives us over to our enemies.

Study Unit Nine:
Spiritual Blocks to Healing

See *A More Excellent Way*™, 7th Edition, pages 253 – 316*

You may have done the 8 Rs and you still have not been healed. Sometimes just discerning and repenting, renouncing, taking responsibility and resisting does not result in healing. The blocks to healing are just as important as the spiritual roots of disease.

Your healing may be blocked because of a lack of sanctification in a certain area of your life. There has to be a heart change on the inside. After you have repented and renounced and resisted, God may need to sanctify you in a particular area of your existence.

- **Healing and deliverance** come as a direct result of sanctification.

- **Disease prevention** can also be a direct result of sanctification.

Sustaining Grace and Greater Grace

There is the traditional, fundamentalist position that says God's grace is sufficient for us.

And he said unto me, My grace is sufficient for thee: for my strength is made perfect in weakness. Most gladly therefore will I rather

---

* Page numbers refer to *A More Excellent Way*™

glory in my infirmities, that the power of Christ may rest upon me.   2 Corinthians 12:9

Sustaining grace is His provision of grace and mercy in our lives at all times, including in the midst of the problem. However, there is a greater grace which is the total absence of the problem. God gets all the glory in this grace.

> **¹¹And God wrought special miracles by the hands of Paul:**
> **¹²So that from his body were brought unto the sick handkerchiefs or aprons, and the diseases departed from them, and the evil spirits went out of them.**   Acts 19:11-12

> **⁸And it came to pass, that the father of Publius lay sick of a fever and of a bloody flux: to whom Paul entered in, and prayed, and laid his hands on him, and healed him.**
> **⁹So when this was done, others also, which had diseases in the island, came, and were healed:**   Acts 28:8-9

1. Do you think that sustaining grace includes us when we are in our problems as well as out of our problems?   yes ___ no ___

2. Is the greater grace "a more excellent way" than sustaining grace?   yes ___ no ___

God meets all of us, regardless of who we are and our circumstances in this journey as pilgrims. You and I are pilgrims, called by God, called by His name and sealed by His Spirit. We are not as we shall be, but in a twinkling of an eye we shall be changed.

So, our hope is in the redemption of our souls and our bodies and the establishment of the kingdom of God in righteousness on this planet. One day you and I will partake of that glorious promise that God through Jesus Christ has given us.

Regardless of the curse? Yes.
Regardless of the fall of Adam? Yes.
Regardless of Satan and sin? Yes.

You may know the roots of your disease, but that is no guarantee that you will be healed. Even though you know the roots of the disease, there may be blocks that prevent God from moving in your life.

3.   Isaiah 5:13 says,
      My people have gone into captivity because they have no _____.

4.   Hosea 4:6 says,
      My people perish for lack of _____.

Discernment opens the door to understanding. It brings us to a place where we observe the spiritual principles of good and evil.

5.   Hebrew 5:14 says,
      But strong meat belongeth to them that are of full age, even those who by reason of use have their senses exercised to _____ both good and evil.

This scripture says that when we have spiritual maturity, it allows us to take a look at all things and judge all things on the basis of discernment. However, discernment alone does not produce freedom, because there may be blocks to healing.

Have you read in the Bible those words: "if, then and but?" In many scriptures there are conditions for receiving God's promises. His promises are all "yea and amen," *but* we first have to *appropriate* them through our *obedience*.

First Samuel 15:22-24 says:

> ²²And Samuel said, Hath the LORD as great delight in burnt offerings and sacrifices, as in obeying the voice of the LORD? Behold, to obey is better than sacrifice, and to hearken than the fat of rams.
> ²³For rebellion is as the sin of witchcraft, and stubbornness is as iniquity and idolatry. Because thou hast rejected the word of the LORD, he hath also rejected thee from being king.
> ²⁴And Saul said unto Samuel, I have sinned: for I have transgressed the commandment of the LORD, and thy words: because I feared the people, and obeyed their voice.   1 Samuel 15:22-24

We need to come to a place where we keep His commandments because we love him.

If ye love me, keep my commandments.
John 14:15

There are examples in the Word that show how God's grace extends beyond His judgments and that He gives us a measure of time that we may apply our hearts to righteousness to get this thing figured out. We see that even under the law, grace and mercy was a factor of God's nature.

However, grace and mercy do not negate our responsibility for obedience to the living God and His

Word. I *know* that I *have* to obey His commandments, but under the covenant of grace and mercy:

- I do not do it because the law requires it.
- I do it because I love God and I love the Lord Jesus.

**Isn't it a small thing for you
to be obedient
to the One you love?**

The enemy does not have the right to afflict you just because he wants to. There must be *open doors* in your family tree or in your personal life, or both, in which you have wandered outside the parameters of God's knowledge, His provision and His covenant.

**As the bird by wandering, as the swallow by
flying, so the curse causeless shall not come.**
Proverbs 26:2

What are open doors? Some diseases have a right to be in our lives because somewhere along the way we, or our ancestors, opened the door to them through sin.

Satan does not have the right to arbitrarily afflict us. If he did, he would have already eliminated the body of Christ worldwide. Since that has not happened, it indicates that the same parameters of protection are here today as were there in the days of Job.

Job had some open doors that allowed him to be sifted by the devil. Bitterness, fear, arrogance and spiritual pride were open doors in Job's life, but he got the message. When he did, God restored to him double what he had lost. page 257

Job had sins in his life, which revealed he was separated from God in several areas. Separation from God in an area would be a block to receiving healing. These blocks are very common to all men, including Christians, and they hinder us from fully walking in the Spirit and receiving the blessings of God.

If you find that you have a block to healing, repent for it and allow your heart to be changed in that area. Do this in the same way you would remove a spiritual root after recognizing it. Use the 8 Rs to freedom.

1) Unforgiveness

2) Ignorance or Lack of Knowledge

3) No Relationship with God According to Knowledge

4) Personal and Family Sins

5) Not Having Faith in God

6) The Need to See a Miracle

7) Looking for Signs and Wonders

8) Expecting God to Heal on One's Own Terms

9) Looking to Man Rather Than God

10) Not Being Honest and Transparent

11) Flagrant Sin or Habitual Sin

12) Robbing God in Tithes and Offerings

13) Some are Just Not Saved

14) Sin of Our Parents

15) Sometimes the Sickness is Unto Death

16) Our Allotted Time in Life is Fulfilled

17) Looking to Symptoms and not to the Healer

18) Letting Fear Enter your Heart

19) Failure to get away in Prayer and Fasting

20) Improper Care of the Body

21) Not Discerning the Lord's Body

22) Touching God's Anointed Leaders

23) Immoderate Eating

24) Pure Unbelief

25) Failing to Keep our Life Filled up with God

26) Not Resisting the Enemy

27) Just Giving Up

28) Looking for Repeated Healings Instead of Divine Health

29) Rejecting Healing as a Part of the Covenant Today

30) Trying to Bypass the Penalty of the Curse

31) Murmuring and Complaining

32) Hating and not Obeying Instruction

33) Past and Continued Involvement with Occultism

1) Underline Unforgiveness

If we refuse to forgive,
we are wasting our time even talking to God
on the subject of healing.

When you read Mark 11:25-26, there is a *conditional* scripture attached.

6.   Mark 11:25-26 says,

    25And when ye stand praying, _____, if ye have ought against any: that your Father also which is in heaven may _____ you your trespasses.

    26But if ye do not forgive, neither will your Father which is in heaven _____ your trespasses.

God's forgiveness for you
is in direct relationship
to how you forgive your brother.

Forgiveness from the Father
is not a one-way street.

Who is it that gives you
a high-octane ping in your spirit
when their name comes up
or when you face them?

If a person is dead,
can you correct the wrong with that person?
No. But you can change the attitude
of your heart toward him or her.
What about people who refuse

to interact with you?
What about someone
you do not know how to contact?

If you have a forgiveness issue
from your past and it is not possible
for you to make it right with the person,
then sincerely make it right with God.

Does this change anything?
When you do this,
you do not have to carry the guilt
about this issue any longer.

You are going to have to make peace in your heart with every person that you have ever known, and get that resolved before God.

> **Whose soever sins ye remit, they are remitted unto them; and whose soever sins ye retain, they are retained.** John 20:23

A big spiritual block to forgiveness occurs when someone sins against us, and we make the sin *equal* to the person. This is a problem because when we make the sin equal to the person, we are not only having a perfect hatred of sin, we are also having a perfect hatred for the person who is in the sin.

When God saved you,
He separated you from your sin.
He saw your sin, but He saw you without it,
as described in Ephesians 1:3-6.

Ask yourself:
Do I wait until I feel like it
to forgive some people?
Do I forgive them
because I am obedient to Christ
and His commandments?
Do I do it because it is the law,
or do I do it because that's just the way I am?

The Spirit of God dwelling in you gives you the ability to:

Think like your Father.
Act like your Father.
Talk like your Father.
Forgive like your Father,
whether you feel like it or not.

Does God wait until He feels like it to forgive?
Do you think Jesus felt like forgiving
while He was on the cross?
Make up your mind once and for all
that you are going to forgive
all men
of all manner of sin.

2) Ignorance or Lack of Knowledge

Both Isaiah 5:13 and Hosea 4:6-7 tell us that we have gone into captivity, and are being destroyed because of lack of knowledge.

7.   You cannot have wisdom if you do not preface it with _____.

Ignorance is also a form of knowledge. The problem is that sometimes we are ignorant, and we don't even know it.

Corinthians says,

> For now we see through a glass darkly but then face to face: now I know in part; but then shall I know even as also I am known.
> 1 Corinthians 13:12

3) No Relationship with God According to Knowledge

There is a difference between "lack of knowledge" and "no relationship with God according to knowledge." In our relationship with God, we can come to a place where we are *not meeting Him according to Scripture.*

The Syrophoenician woman in Mark 7:24-30 asked Jesus to cast a devil out of her daughter. Jesus told her that she did not qualify, that she was not in covenant, that she was not with God according to knowledge, that she was outside and separated from God, and that she was asking for something that did not belong to her.

She answered,

> ²⁸...Yes Lord: yet the dogs under the table eat of the children's crumbs.
> ²⁹And He said unto her, For this saying go thy way; the devil is gone out of thy daughter.
> ³⁰And when she was come to her house, she found the devil gone out, and her daughter laid upon the bed. Mark 7:28-30

*Does this story tell us
that you can be healed
without being in covenant?*

*If you are healed or seeking healing
and you are outside of covenant with God,
would it behoove you
to get into covenant quickly?*

*He who has healed you
is He whom you should follow
the rest of your days.*

Get right with God now, because there is no provision for getting saved after you die. There is no stopping-off point or reincarnation facility, only judgment.

> And as it is appointed unto men once to die, but after this the judgment: Hebrews 9:27

Sometimes people do not receive from God, because they do not have a relationship with God according to knowledge. Both the Old and New Testament tell us this.

In Hebrews it says that you must believe that God "is," and that He is a rewarder of them that diligently seek Him.

> ...he that cometh to God must believe that he is, and that he is a rewarder of them that diligently seek him.　　　Hebrews 11:6

> Ye ask, and receive not, <u>because ye ask amiss,</u> that ye may consume *it* upon your lusts.
> 　　　James 4:3

Asking amiss refers to a prayer of *vanity*. God is not interested in answering this type of prayer. He is not interested in answering prayers that are fraudulent.

In Mark 7:6 Jesus said, "Well hath Esaias prophesied of you hypocrites, as it is written, This people honoureth me with their lips, but their heart is far from me." Jesus is referring back to Isaiah 29:13.

> Wherefore the Lord said, Forasmuch as this people draw near me with their mouth, and with their lips do honour me, but have removed their heart far from me, and their fear toward me is taught by the precept of men:　　　Isaiah 29:13

8.　Matthew 6:33 says,
　　Seek ye first the _____ of God and His _____, and all these things shall be added onto you.

Three Phases of Seeking after God

Seeking after God according to knowledge means pursuing relationship with Him. There are three phases of seeking after God according to knowledge.

Fellowship. The first phase of relationship is fellowship with our Creator. Fellowship involves talking to God. It involves having conversation with God about the desires, plans and purposes of *His* heart, not just your heart.

9. James 4:8 says,
    Draw _____to God, and He will draw
    _____to you.

Worship comes next. When you are in fellowship, then you will be in worship.

> But the hour cometh, and now is, when the true worshippers shall worship the Father in spirit and in truth: for the Father seeketh such to worship him.   John 4:23

Petition. Last comes petition. If you come to petition first before you come to fellowship and worship, your petition is fraudulent. It is not according to knowledge. Put what YOU want last.

> *The first thing you have to do is approach God because of WHO He is...*
> *and what He has done for you*
> *from the foundation of the world,*
> *whether He gives you anything or not.*

The gift of salvation is enough. The rest of it is just icing on the cake, but the *foundation* is *salvation*. Some people do not want the Father or the Holy Spirit. They just want the "fix."

Sometimes the attitude of our heart

is a hindrance to our healing.

We approach God according to knowledge on the basis of what we can *prove* in Scripture. Approaching God on the basis of what religion has said, or what man has said, can result in "No relationship with God according to knowledge."

4) Personal and Family Sins

Isaiah says that our sins can separate us from our God. Not only our sins, but also the consequence of our ancestors' iniquities and sins can transfer into us and separate us from God.

> ¹Behold, the LORD'S hand is not shortened, that it cannot save; neither his ear heavy, that it cannot hear:
> ²But your iniquities have separated between you and your God, and your sins have hid *his* face from you, that he will not hear.   Isaiah 59:1-2

Exodus 20:5 adds that the iniquities of the fathers shall be visited upon the children, down to the third and fourth generations. God holds the fathers responsible for the spirituality of the family.

> Thou shalt not bow down thyself to them, nor serve them: for I the LORD thy God *am* a jealous God, visiting the iniquity of the fathers upon the children unto the third and fourth *generation* of them that hate me;   Exodus 20:5

Deuteronomy says it again, exactly the same way.

> Thou shalt not bow down thyself unto them, nor serve them: for I the LORD thy God *am* a jealous God, visiting the iniquity of the fathers

upon the children unto the third and fourth
generation of them that hate me, Deuteronomy 5:9

In Nehemiah 8:1-9:2, you find that Ezra, the
priest and scribe, called all the people together. After
they heard the Word of God for six hours, they
worshipped and confessed their sins and the sins and
iniquities of their fathers before God.

They confessed the sins and iniquities of their
fathers so they could be freed from the curse of sin
coming out of their generations. Look at the attitude of
their hearts:

> ¹And all the people gathered themselves
> together as one man ... and they spake unto Ezra
> the scribe to bring the book of the law of Moses,
> which the LORD had commanded to Israel.
> ²And Ezra the priest brought the law before
> the congregation both of men and women, and
> all that could hear with understanding...
> ³And he read therein before the street that
> *was* before the water gate from the morning
> until midday, before the men and the women,
> and those that could understand; and the ears of
> all the people *were attentive* unto the book of
> the law.
> ⁶And Ezra blessed the LORD, the great God.
> And all the people answered, Amen, Amen, with
> lifting up their hands: and they bowed their
> heads, and worshipped the LORD with *their*
> faces to the ground.
> ⁸So they read in the book in the law of God
> distinctly, and gave the sense, and caused *them*
> to understand the reading.
> ⁹And Nehemiah, which *is* the Tirshatha, and
> Ezra the priest the scribe, and the Levites that
> taught the people, said unto all the people, This
> day *is* holy unto the LORD your God; mourn
> not, nor weep. For all the people wept, when
> they heard the words of the law.

¹⁰... for *this* day *is* holy unto our Lord: neither be ye sorry; for the joy of the LORD is your strength.

¹¹So the Levites stilled all the people, saying, Hold your peace, for the day *is* holy; neither be ye grieved.

¹²And all the people went their way to eat, and to drink, and to send portions, and to make great mirth, because they had understood the words that were declared unto them.

¹³And on the second day were gathered together the chief of the fathers of all the people, the priests, and the Levites, unto Ezra the scribe, even to understand the words of the law.

Nehemiah 8:1-3, 6, 8-13

¹Now in the twenty and fourth day of this month the children of Israel were assembled with fasting, and with sackclothes, and earth upon them.

²And the seed of Israel separated themselves from all strangers, and stood and confessed their sins, and the iniquities of their fathers.

Nehemiah 9:1-2

Can you see evidence that the curse of the fathers is still here today?

Not only do we have to consider personal sins that separate us from our God, we also have to consider generational iniquities that we have inherited through our family tree.

Can you see the bondage and the disease that follow family trees? Can you see personality quirks, dispositional characteristics and even insanity being passed down?

How are we able to see this?
We can see this through simple observation of family trees
and by what the Word says about generational curses
that flow from family to family.

Refer to the Family Health Tree in Unit Two.

5) <u>Not Having Faith in God</u>

What did Jesus say about faith? What is faith?

> **And Jesus answering saith unto them, Have faith in God.** Mark 11:22

> **But without faith *it is* impossible to please *him*: for he that cometh to God must believe that he is, and *that* he is a rewarder of them that diligently seek him.** Hebrews 11:6

> **Now faith is the substance of things hoped for, the evidence of things not seen.** Hebrews 11:1

10. Hebrews 4 says the children of Israel, coming out of Egypt under the leadership of Moses and Aaron, did not enter into promise because of _____ and unbelief.

> **²For unto us was the gospel preached, as well as unto them: but the word preached did not profit them, not being mixed with faith in them that heard *it*...**
> **⁶Seeing therefore it remaineth that some must enter therein, and they to whom it was first preached entered not in because of unbelief:**
> Hebrews 4:2,6

11. When Jesus went back to His hometown of Nazareth, Scripture says He did no great miracles in Nazareth because great was their doubt and _____.

> ⁵And he could there do no mighty work, save
> that he laid his hands upon a few sick folk, and
> healed *them.*
> ⁶And he marvelled because of their unbelief.
> And he went round about the villages, teaching.
>
> Mark 6:5-6

In Mark 5:36-42, Jesus was about to raise a young lady from the dead, and there were a lot of people around because she had died. They were ready to have a wake, and He walked in and said, "But she's just sleeping." They laughed at Him and scorned Him.

Jesus put them out of the room, brought the family and His disciples into the room, and He raised her from the dead. He put them out of the room because their unbelief and doubt would negate His power and ability to heal.

What happens when there is doubt and unbelief in your heart?

Pastor Henry says, "If there is unbelief and doubt in your heart concerning me as a pastor, I would stagger under it. I would only be able to do a few things for you. Will you mix your faith with mine before God?"

As we come into agreement and mix our faith together before God, we are trusting Him to honor us. We are trusting Him to convict us. We trust Him to work with us. We ask Him, in faith, to come to us.

> I tell you that he will avenge them speedily.
> Nevertheless when the Son of man cometh, shall
> he find faith on the earth? Luke 18:8

6) The Need to See a Miracle

Many people will not believe until they have seen a miracle.

Those who mocked Jesus on the cross

Regarding Jesus on the cross, Matthew says,

> ³⁹And they that passed by reviled Him, wagging their heads,
> ⁴⁰And saying, Thou that destroyest the temple and buildest it in three days, save Thyself. If Thou be the Son of God, come down from the cross.   Matthew 27:39-40

They wanted to see a miracle before they would believe. They wanted to see Jesus come off the cross, but if He had, you and I wouldn't be here today.

Peter

When Jesus was preparing the disciples for His crucifixion, He told them that He would go to Jerusalem and that He would be betrayed and be crucified. Peter rebuked Him and kind of "told Him off."

Jesus responded to Peter. He said, "Get behind me, Satan."

Thomas

Thomas said he wouldn't believe Jesus was raised from the dead until he saw the scars, so Jesus showed him the scars in His hands and in His side.

> ²⁷Then saith he to Thomas, Reach hither thy finger, and behold my hands; and reach hither thy hand, and thrust *it* into my side: and be not faithless, but believing.

²⁸And Thomas answered and said unto him, My Lord and my God.

²⁹Jesus saith unto him, Thomas, because thou hast seen me, thou hast believed: blessed *are* they that have not seen, and *yet* have believed.

John 20:27-29

Temptation of Christ by Satan

Look at how Satan tempted our LORD Jesus in this area.

¹Then was Jesus led up of the Spirit into the wilderness to be tempted of the devil.

²And when he had fasted forty days and forty nights, he was afterward an hungred.

³And when the tempter came to him, he said, If thou be the Son of God, command that these stones be made bread.   Matthew 4:1-3

Satan was saying, "Do something."

When you look at me, Henry Wright, as a Pastor:

"If you do not see God and the sanctifying work of the Word behind me, you have a block. If I do not become invisible so that all you see is *Him*, you have a block. All I am is His slave and His servant."

You are to look to *Him*, to the sanctifying work of the Holy Spirit and to the Word of God.

Have you asked God to do something for you?
Have you put out a fleece, saying,
"God, if You will do this, then I will believe You?"

Could you just believe Him to begin with?
If He wants to do something for you,
wouldn't He just do it?

How?
He would come to you
and deal with you in the areas
where you are separated from Him,
so that He could bless you with the desire of your heart.

7) Looking for Signs and Wonders

If we seek God and His Word as the foundation of our faith, then signs and wonders will chase after us!

There is a difference between chasing signs and wonders
and having signs and wonders follow you.

The key is to have faith in God and His Word
on the basis of relationship,
not on the basis of signs and manifestations.

Some people are looking for signs, rather than the Word of God. In Cana, a man asked Jesus to heal his son. In John 4:46-48, Jesus told him "…Except ye see signs and wonders, ye will not believe."

Matthew says,

> [38]Then certain of the scribes and of the Pharisees answered, saying, Master, we would see a sign from thee.
>
> [39]But he answered and said unto them, An evil and adulterous generation seeketh after a sign; and there shall no sign be given to it, but the sign of the prophet Jonas: Matthew 12:38-39

8) Expecting God to Heal on One's Own Terms

Some people expect God to heal them on their own terms. They tell God exactly what to do, when to do it, and how to do it.

The Example of Naaman — 2 Kings 5:8-14

Naaman was an important individual. He was the captain of the host of the king of Syria...a great and honorable man. He was of great value to his master, and he had leprosy. He came a great distance to find Elisha, the man of God who he had heard could heal him or fix him and get him right.

> [10]And Elisha sent a messenger unto him, saying, Go and wash in the Jordan seven times, and thy flesh shall come again to thee, and thou shalt be clean.
>
> [11]But Naaman was wroth, and went away, and said, Behold, I thought, He will surely come out to me, and stand, and call on the name of the LORD his God, and strike his hand over the place, and recover the leper.
>
> [12]*Are* not Abana and Pharpar, rivers of Damascus, better than all the waters of Israel? may I not wash in them, and be clean? So he turned and went away in a rage.   2 Kings 5:10-12

You can see Naaman's pride in verse 11. He had already figured out how it was going to go. However, Elisha didn't go meet him at all. He sent his servant. That takes care of idolatry, doesn't it? You have to be careful that you don't make your spiritual leaders an icon. Be careful that you don't make those who rule over you greater than they really are. God is no respecter of persons.

> ...of a truth I perceive that God is no respecter of persons: Acts 10:34

What did Elisha tell the messenger to say? Go down to the river and wash seven times. What was Naaman's reaction? "What? You do not know who you are talking to. I want Elisha to come out here and call unto his God in heaven, and strike his hand over the place. I want to see a miracle."

Sometimes we expect God to heal us on our own terms in the way that we think it should happen.

Naaman had spiritual problems. He was dealing with spiritual roots of pride, bitterness, resentment, unforgiveness, rage and anger.

> [13]And his servants came near, and spake unto him, and said, My father, *if* the prophet had bid thee *do some* great thing, wouldest thou not have done *it*? how much rather then, when he saith to thee, Wash, and be clean? 2 Kings 5:13

Who had the wisdom for the matter? His servants! Did he respond to them? Yes. Did he get healed? Yes.

> Then went he down, and dipped himself
> seven times in Jordan, according to the saying of
> the man of God: and his flesh came again like
> unto the flesh of a little child, and he was clean.
>
> 2 Kings 5:14

9) Looking to Man Rather Than God

This ministry is not against physicians or psychiatrists, but they are not qualified to deal with the spiritual roots of disease to bring forth healing, and the church has negated its role in the healing of disease by asking doctors to become spiritual healers.

However, born again believers are the ones who are qualified. We know this from the Word. The gifts of healing are given by the Holy Spirit in 1 Corinthians 12:8-10.

> [8]For to one is given by the Spirit the word of
> wisdom; to another the word of knowledge by
> the same Spirit;
> [9]To another faith by the same Spirit; to
> another the gifts of healing by the same Spirit;
> [10]To another the working of miracles; to
> another prophecy; to another discerning of
> spirits; to another *divers* kinds of tongues; to
> another the interpretation of tongues:
>
> 1 Corinthians 12:8-10

Ephesians says,

> [11]And he gave some, apostles; and some,
> prophets; and some, evangelists; and some,
> pastors and teachers;
> [12]For the perfecting of the saints, for the work
> of the ministry, for the edifying of the body of
> Christ:
>
> Ephesians 4:11-12

According to these scriptures, are doctors qualified to heal you of spiritually rooted diseases? No! Are they listed in the fivefold ministry giftings of Ephesians 4? No! Who has been ordained to heal? God has ordained the church to be involved in healing the body.

Doctors can only offer disease management, in cases where a disease is spiritually rooted. However, it is not wrong to go to a doctor to get a diagnosis for the problem, to find out what is going on. We recommend that you do, because we do not play games with people's lives. We meet people where they are, as they come to us each day.

As born again believers, what we really need are doctors who understand that there are spiritual components to disease and who will work with pastors. Pastors should also have a better understanding of the role of the church in the healing of disease.

The Example of Asa — 2 Chronicles 16:7-12

Asa died. One of the reasons he died was because he did not seek the LORD first, not only in war, but also in his personal life. God had already proven Himself to be on Asa's side in previous wars. Asa's heart had hardened in his apostasy and in his darkness, and he had a disease that was unto death.

> And Asa in the thirty and ninth year of his reign was diseased in his feet, until his disease was exceeding great: yet in his disease he sought not to the LORD, but to the physicians.
>
> 2 Chronicles 16:12

If we continue to look to doctors for healing *before* seeking God, without giving consideration to the spiritual dynamics behind the curse of disease, this is also a block to healing. In Asa's case, it caused his death.

Jeremiah says,

> ⁵Thus saith the Lord; Cursed be the man that trusteth in man, and maketh flesh his arm, and whose heart departeth from the Lord...
> ⁶Blessed is the man that trusteth in the LORD, and whose hope the Lord is...
>
> Jeremiah 17:5-6

One of the great blocks
to receiving healing from God
is looking to man to be your source.

Have you ever looked to man
as your source rather than to God?
If so, repent and turn to Him.

At this level, the church has failed in its mission to represent God. Many churches teach their people to believe in God, but they do not understand disease and the cause for it. In 80 percent of all cases, disease has a spiritual root. The people have nowhere to turn except to man, because the church has negated its role in the healing of spiritually rooted disease.

10) <u>Not Being Honest and Transparent</u>

Two main reasons for not being honest and transparent are fear and pride. Fear of rejection, fear of man, fear of failure, fear of abandonment and fear of not being loved cause us to cover up who we really are.

Pride is very dangerous because it can make you appear holy when you are not. It produces an existence that is fraudulent. In other words, you are living a lie. It's a high price to pay, because it produces a fall and also much disease.

> Pride goeth before destruction, and an haughty spirit before a fall. Proverbs 16:18

Did you forget that God sees you?
Did you forget that God already knows everything?
Do you think you are hiding anything from God?
He knows my thoughts, and He knows your thoughts.

James 5:16 tells us to confess our faults one to another, that we may be healed. Galatians 6:1 tells us how we are instructed to respond in meekness towards someone who has fallen into sin.

The book of Proverbs says,

> He that covereth his sins shall not prosper: but whosoever confesseth and forsaketh them shall have mercy. Proverbs 28:13

Isaiah said it this way,

> For thus saith the high and lofty One that inhabiteth eternity...I dwell in the high and holy place, with him also that is of a contrite and humble spirit. Isaiah 57:15

Can we trust each other?
Is it safe to be honest and transparent?

Being honest and transparent
should be safe for believers,
because perfect love covers a multitude of sins.

And above all things have fervent charity
among yourselves: for charity shall cover the
multitude of sins.   1 Peter 4:8

There is no fear in love; but perfect love
casteth out fear: because fear hath torment. He
that feareth is not made perfect in love.
                                            1 John 4:18

11) Flagrant Sin or Habitual Sin

There is a difference between (1) temptation, (2)
falling into sin then repenting and getting out of sin,
and (3) living habitually in sin.

Temptation is not the same as sin. Jesus was
tempted in all points such as we are, yet was without
sin. So we know that temptation is not sin.

For we have not an high priest which cannot
be touched with the feeling of our infirmities;
but was in all points tempted like as *we are, yet*
without sin.   Hebrews 4:15

Paul uses Galatians 5:19-21 to defeat legalism
and to establish our freedom from legalism.

19Now the works of the flesh are manifest,
which   are   these;   Adultery,   fornication,
uncleanness, lasciviousness,

²⁰Idolatry, witchcraft, hatred, variance, emulations, wrath, strife, seditions, heresies,

²¹Envyings, murders, drunkenness, revellings, and such like: of the which I tell you before, as I have also told you in time past, that they which do such things shall not inherit the kingdom of God.   Galatians 5:19-21

In verse 21, the word "do" refers to those who *habitually* practice those things against God with a hardened heart as a way of life... It is important to understand that grace and mercy do not absolve us from responsibility for holiness.

*Have you been exposed to teachings
that remove responsibility for sin
because of grace and mercy?*

*Do you understand the Word says
that the wages of sin is still death?
(Romans 6:23)*

*Do you believe that there are still consequences
to sin in the New Covenant?
Do you see psychological and biological diseases
engulfing the Christian church?*

*Deuteronomy 28 clearly states that all disease
is a result of separation from God,
and disobedience to His Word.*

*Since we know that God does not condone sin in our lives,
why is it that grace and mercy
seem to be extended to one person
and not the other?*

12. The person who is not accepted before God has a heart that is _____ toward God. This person does not have any desire to change.

13. But the other person has, because of temptation, fallen into sin, but has a perfect _____ for it. So even though he is still in bondage, his heart is right before God against the sin. God is dealing with that person and working him over.

It is not the sin itself. God looks at the attitude of your heart toward the sin.

12) Robbing God in Tithes and Offerings

Malachi 3:8-11 tells about robbing God in our tithes and offerings.

14. Why were the people of God cursed with a curse according to Malachi 3? Because they had not brought their _____ and _____into the storehouse.

This is considered robbing God because everything you have belongs to Him, even your paycheck. Your paycheck is also God's. He's just loaning it to you.

The Bible says that you are not working for an employer; you are working for the Lord. Even if he or she is unjust, you are still working for the Lord.

It is possible to rob other things from God besides money. Robbing God is not just in tithes and offerings, but also in the "firstfruits" of our substance, including our time. The best belongs to God.

Honor the LORD with thy substance, and
with the firstfruits of all thine increase:

Proverbs 3:9

13) Some Are Just Not Saved

Sometimes people will stay in their disease and
perish because they do not receive the truth that would
save them. They do not know Jesus or the Father.

10...they received not the love of the truth,
that they might be saved.
11And for this cause God shall send them
strong delusion, that they should believe a lie:

2 Thessalonians 2:10-11

That scripture is saying that if you want to
believe error, God will allow more error to come into
your life.

14) Sin of Our Parents

In 2 Samuel chapters 11-12, you can read the
story of the adulterous affair that David had with
Bathsheba. In chapter 12, verses 13-14, it talks about the
curse of death on David and Bathsheba's child. The
child died because of the sins of adultery and murder
in the lives of the parents.

Howbeit, because by this deed thou hast
given great occasion to the enemies of the LORD
to blaspheme, the child also that is born unto
thee shall surely die.   2 Samuel 12:14

David's actions gave the enemy an advantage.
Our words and our actions give the enemy an
opportunity to blaspheme.

*Do you think about
how your words and actions
give your enemies a reason
to blaspheme the Lord?*

David confesses to God in Psalm 51. He says,

**Against thee, thee only, have I sinned, and
done this evil in thy sight...** Psalm 51:4

When we sin, we do evil towards God.

In 1 Kings 14:1-13, there is a tremendous statement about God taking a child in death. This is the only scripture Pastor Wright has found where God has taken anyone through a disease just to preserve that person for Himself.

God knew if the child were allowed to live, his evil parents would pervert his heart; and if that happened, He would lose him forever, so He took the child in disease to preserve him in the resurrection.

That is a valuable insight that can help you understand more about the people who die in disease. Sometimes we don't understand and have to let God be sovereign, knowing His ways are higher than our ways.

15) Sometimes the Sickness is Unto Death

Second Chronicles 21:4-20 tells the story of Jehoram. He was a man that once knew God, but he turned away from Him.

He killed his brothers, and because of murder he got sick and died. The Bible says he committed a sin unto death.

There are certain sins unto death that cause people to die from disease.

First John 5:16, talks about a sin unto death. John says in this verse, "I would not that you pray for it."

> ¹⁶If any man see his brother sin a sin *which is not unto death*, he shall ask, and he shall give him life for them that sin not unto death. There is a sin unto death: I do not say that he shall pray for it.
> ¹⁷All unrighteousness is sin: and there is a sin not unto death.   1 John 5:16-17

Second Kings 1:2-8 is the story of Ahaziah. He dabbled in sorcery. Under the law of Moses, sorcery, witchcraft and occultism brought a penalty of death. Ahaziah died because his sin was unto death.

King Saul died prematurely because of his sins. Saul disobeyed God, and he contacted the witch of Endor who had a familiar spirit. When Saul committed suicide, he was judged in death because he disobeyed God and because he consulted with a familiar spirit. (1 Chronicles 10:14)

Occultism is the spiritual root of many diseases unto death.

In His first commandment, God said, "You shall have no other gods before Me." Involvement in occultism can open the door to a spirit of death and bring a curse of many diseases.

214

*How do we know what kind of sin to pray for,
and what kind of sin not to pray for?*

*If I see you in sin
that will not produce a disease
that will kill you,
then I shall pray to God for you that He may heal you.*

*But if I see you in sin
that produces a disease unto death,
I shall not pray for you
until the sin issue is dealt with,
because it is a sin that is unto death.*

Many diseases we deal with are spiritually rooted and are diseases unto death. Diseases coming out of bitterness and unforgiveness are examples of this. Cancer is a disease unto death that comes out of bitterness. Diabetes is a death disease coming right out of self-hatred.

If a disease is unto death, you are wasting time praying for it until the sin issues are dealt with. Get involved in the people's lives. Tell them that according to the Word of God you cannot pray for them until the sin issues are dealt with. Deal with the sin issue first, then pray and minister. (See 2 Timothy 2:24-26 and Galatians 6:1.)

Jesus healed every single person that came to Him. That isn't happening today, because something is missing. Sanctification for healing is the dimension that is missing from teachings in the churches today.

We need to teach sanctification and bring people to a place of repentance for their sin. If I ask God to heal you while you continue in your sin, I would be asking Him to dishonor His Word by condoning your sin.

16) Our Allotted Time in Life is Fulfilled

In Psalm 90, by His Spirit through Moses, God established the longevity of man as threescore and ten, which is seventy comfortable years; or fourscore, which is eighty years with "some trouble." Anything less than 70 to 80 years of longevity on this planet is a curse.

God's promise is that we should have longevity in order to establish His righteousness in our generation, and that we may number our days in righteousness and be part of His plan, His kingdom.

When you find men whose lives were cut short,
you will see a curse attached to it.

17) Looking to Symptoms and Not to the Healer

²⁸And Peter answered him and said, Lord, if it be thou, bid me come unto thee on the water.

²⁹And he said, Come. And when Peter was come down out of the ship, he walked on the water, to go to Jesus.

³⁰But when he saw the wind boisterous, he was afraid; and beginning to sink, he cried, saying, Lord, save me.   Matthew 14:28-30

As long as Peter kept his eyes on the Lord, he was fine. When he took his eyes off of the LORD, he went into *unbelief* and started to sink.

Are we going into unbelief
when we are looking at the symptoms
of our disease instead of God?

Get your eyes off your pain.
Get your eyes off your disease.
Get your eyes back on the LORD
and His Word and keep them there.

The symptoms of your disease
are the fruit of your problem.
The symptoms are not the root.

The book of Proverbs says,

The spirit of a man will sustain his infirmity; but a wounded spirit who can bear?
Proverbs 18:14

Scripture teaches that we are seated with Christ Jesus in heavenly places, far above all principalities and powers. We should walk in the Spirit. (See Ephesians 1:19-23, Ephesians 2:6 and Romans 8:11.) page 293

217

As you stand before Him,
ask for His mercy
concerning the roots and blocks
of your disease.

Remember who you are
and where you are in the battle.
You are born again,
a new creature in Christ.

Remember that you are
more than a physical body.
Keep your eyes off the symptoms
and on the Lord.
Your spirit must be alive to God.

18) Letting Fear Enter Your Heart

God has something to say about the spirit of fear
in His Word.

15. Romans 8:15 says,
    > For ye have not received the spirit of bondage
    > again to _____; but ye have received the Spirit
    > of adoption, whereby we cry, Abba, Father.

16. Romans 14:23 says,
    > ...for whatsoever is not of _____ is sin.

17. John 14:1 says,
    > Let not your heart be_____: ye believe in
    > God, believe also in me.

What will fear do to you?
Fear will quench your faith.
What quenches fear?
Faith will quench your fears.

You can choose which will rule you.
Faith and fear are equal in this dimension.
Both demand to be fulfilled,
and both project into the future.

18. Hebrews 11:1 says,
> Now faith is the substance of things
> _____ for, the evidence of things not seen.
> Fear is also the substance of things_____ for, the evidence of things not yet seen.

19) Failure to Get Away in Prayer and Fasting

Many people believe that we pray and fast to *receive* from God. Actually, we should pray and fast to *meet* God in relationship. There is a lot of confusion, because there is more than one kind of fast unto the LORD, and their purposes are different.

Isaiah 58 shows a different kind of fast. It is not a fast from food and water. This fast has to do with your service unto God on behalf of others — to both strangers and family.

As you give unto others, God will give back to you.
Serving others breaks the yoke of bondage.

In Matthew 17:18-21, the disciples had to undergo prayer and fasting because they could not cast out the spirit of epilepsy. They had gotten so involved in making a "science" out of this new ministry of healing in Christ, that they forgot they were supposed to be in a tightly knit relationship with the Father and Jesus.

If you do not ever pray and fast,
it will be a block to the hand of God.

Prayer and fasting allows God to enrich you and bring you back to that place of fellowship where He is your priority. You set aside everything, including eating, so as to have a period of time where you are completely alone with God and His Word for relationship purposes.

Prayer and fasting is not for the purpose of getting something from God. Do not confuse petition with fellowship when it comes to prayer and fasting. Prayer and fasting is primarily for fellowship, out of which God blesses us.

20) Improper Care of the Body

God is not going to answer prayers for your healing if you are not getting good nutrition, drinking enough water or getting enough rest and sleep.

Prolonged illness can be the consequence of negligence. Burnout can be another aspect of improper care of the body. In Philippians 2:25-30, there is a story about someone serving the Lord who got sick unto death because he did not use wisdom in how much time he spent in ministry serving the Lord.

21) Not Discerning the Lord's Body

> ²⁹For he that eateth and drinketh unworthily, eateth and drinketh damnation to himself, not discerning the Lord's body.
> ³⁰For this cause many *are* weak and sickly among you, and many sleep.
>
> 1 Corinthians 11:29-30

19. What did Paul say were the consequences of not discerning the LORD'S body? Paul said, "many are _____, and _____ among you and many _____" because they did not discern the LORD's body.

It is the "LORD's body" we must discern. It is by His stripes we were and are healed.

> ⁴Surely he hath borne our griefs, and carried our sorrows: yet we did esteem him stricken, smitten of God, and afflicted.
> ⁵But he *was* wounded for our transgressions, *he was* bruised for our iniquities: the chastisement of our peace *was* upon him; and with his stripes we are healed.   Isaiah 53:4-5

> That it might be fulfilled which was spoken by Esaias the prophet, saying, Himself took our infirmities, and bare *our* sicknesses.   Matthew 8:17

> Who his own self bare our sins in his own body on the tree, that we, being dead to sins, should live unto righteousness: by whose stripes ye were healed.   1 Peter 2:24

You can avoid being weak and sickly and dying a premature death by having faith in the healing and forgiveness that was provided by Christ. With such faith, nothing will be impossible.

20. Mark 11:22-24 says,

> ²²And Jesus answering saith unto them, Have faith in God.
>
> ²³For verily I say unto you, That whosoever shall say unto this mountain, Be thou removed, and be thou cast into the sea; and shall not doubt in his heart, but shall believe that those things which he saith shall come to pass; he shall have whatsoever he saith.
>
> ²⁴Therefore I say unto you, What things soever ye desire, when ye pray, _____that ye receive *them,* and ye shall have *them.*

Communion

First Corinthians chapter 11 tells us about taking communion in unbelief, not realizing its true significance and not discerning the LORD's body and blood to receive the benefits by faith.

It also refers to the saved or unsaved man who takes communion with sin in his life, without making confession unto salvation and acknowledging personal needs, and without judging himself so as to escape the chastening of the God.

> ²⁷Wherefore whosoever shall eat this bread, and drink this cup of the Lord, unworthily, shall be guilty of the body and blood of the Lord.
>
> ²⁸But let a man examine himself, and so let him eat of *that* bread, and drink of *that* cup.
>
> ²⁹For he that eateth and drinketh unworthily, eateth and drinketh damnation to himself, not discerning the Lord's body.

³⁰For this cause many *are* weak and sickly among you, and many sleep.

³¹For if we would judge ourselves, we should not be judged.   1 Corinthians 11:27-31

*If we take communion
without realizing its true significance,
will we receive chastening? Yes!*

*If we take communion
without discerning the Lord's body and blood
to receive the benefits by faith,
will we receive chastening? Yes!*

*If we take communion with sin in our lives,
without making confession unto salvation
and without judging ourselves,
will we receive chastening? Yes!*

*What about the unsaved?
The unsaved man who takes communion
with sin in his life,
without making confession unto salvation,
and without judging himself,
will also receive God's chastening.*

Three Aspects of Not Discerning the Lord's Body

Aspect one is partaking unworthily.

Only three sacraments are found in Scripture as commandments: water baptism, communion and foot washing. In communion you are celebrating the remembrance of Christ in two dimensions: His shed blood and His broken body.

When you unworthily partake of what God's forgiveness represents in communion, *without repenting to Him*, you are guilty of fraud, and you have cursed yourself with a curse. You have cursed yourself with a curse because you make what Jesus did at the cross of no effect for you.

It is not the sacrament that saves you.
It is the obedience.

When we partake unworthily, we *fail to judge ourselves* with regard to sin being the spiritual root of disease. When we judge ourselves, it brings forth repentance so that forgiveness, deliverance and healing can be *appropriated*. This appropriation is what brings forth the full benefit provided in the LORD's Supper.

Judging ourselves involves having the discernment to know specifically what is being repented for. Otherwise we do not know what to stand against, what to change in our lives, and what to renounce in our lives. Many people say, "Father God, forgive me of all my sins," and He does forgive, but there can be no repentance without *specifically* knowing the sin area that needs to be sanctified in our lives.

Aspect two is "Eating each other alive."

This happens when believers in the body attack one another in relationships, as an autoimmune disease attacks the physical body.

The church is the body of Christ.
We must learn to discern one another
as part of one body.

Now ye are the body of Christ, and members
in particular.   1 Corinthians 12:27

Bear ye one another's burdens, and so fulfil
the law of Christ.   Galatians 6:2

Can you love the LORD if you hate your
brother? No. If you say you love the LORD, yet you
hate your brother, the love of God is not with you.

We know that we have passed from death
unto life, because we love the brethren. He that
loveth not *his* brother abideth in death.
                    1 John 3:14

When we partake of communion
in remembrance of Him,
we are saying to Him
that because of what He did for us,
we are ready to do that for each other.

Christ has already laid down His life for us, but
we still need to lay down our lives for each other. We
are not dying for each other's sins, but we are to lay
our lives down in service, one to another.

If we ignore our brother who is in need, then we
have negated that fellowship with him that
communion represents. There is a consequence for
refusing fellowship with each other at that level. If we
are not in fellowship at that level, we are cursed with a
curse (disease).

The word "communion" is *koinonia* (*#2842, Greek, Strong's Concordance*) – fellowship. We must focus on the horizontal relationship in the body of Christ, which is our relationship with each other, as well as on the vertical relationship with each of the three persons of the Godhead.

> [16]The cup of blessing which we bless, is it not the communion of the blood of Christ? The bread which we break, is it not the communion of the body of Christ?
> [17]For we *being* many are one bread, *and* one body: for we are all partakers of that one bread.
> 1 Corinthians 10:16-17

The cup (the blood) represents forgiveness of sins both on the vertical level from God and on the horizontal level toward each other.

The bread represents the bread of life for the healing of our bodies. This comes as the result of us helping one another deal with the spiritual roots of disease and blocks to healing. It is the church being the church, and ministering the life of God to each other.

There are benefits to partaking of this sacrament properly. When we are partaking of communion correctly, then we can truly say:

> For the kingdom of God is not meat and drink; but righteousness, and peace, and joy in the Holy Ghost.　　　　Romans 14:17

Aspect three is not believing that healing is for today.

This third aspect of "not discerning the LORD'S body" as taught in 1 Corinthians 11, is even more serious. It is addressed to churches that do not believe that healing is for today. Many churches do not believe that what was provided for us at the cross is represented by the communion service.

The shed blood of Jesus was not for the *healing* of disease. His shed blood was for the *forgiveness* of sins. Scripture is clear — without the shedding of blood, there is no *remission* of sins.

> For this is my blood of the new testament, which is shed for many for the remission of sins.
> Matthew 26:28

> And almost all things are by the law purged with blood; and without shedding of blood is no remission.
> Hebrews 9:22

When we come into communion and take the cup, we acknowledge that what He did for us allows us to repent, to be cleansed and to be forgiven of all sin (1 John 1:7-10).

21. The broken bread represents the stripes that were laid on Jesus. The bread represents freedom from the curse. The curse includes all manner of _____ (Deuteronomy 28).

> Who his own self bare our sins in his own body on the tree, that we, being dead to sins, should live unto righteousness: by whose stripes ye were healed.
> 1 Peter 2:24

When we take the bread of communion, which represents freedom from the curse, but do not believe that freedom from disease is for today, we bring a curse into our lives.

The curse is the disease that we say we cannot be healed from; while at the same time, we celebrate the sacrament that provides for that healing.

This is not theologically sound. When we do this we negate one-half of what Christ did at the cross. In partaking of the bread unworthily, we curse ourselves in our ignorance and our apostasy.

22) Touching God's Anointed Leaders

There is a major curse that comes with touching God's anointed.

> ...touch not mine anointed, and do my prophets no harm. 1 Chronicles 16:22

> ...touch not mine anointed, and do my prophets no harm. Psalm 105:15

God's anointed are all those set in place in leadership in the church and their families. If you have a pastor that is in error, the elders ought to be able to straighten him out. He is God's servant, and when it's all said and done, God is the One who will deal with him.

Read for yourself in the Bible about Korah and the 250 elders of Israel that went into sedition against Moses in Numbers 16.

Miriam, Moses' sister, was struck with leprosy because of her murmuring against the wife of Moses in Numbers 12.

Words spoken against a pastor affect your health. What you say about your pastor and church leaders is very important to your health and well-being.

People do not understand the seriousness of the sins of the tongue and the sin of division against God's leaders and those who minister under them.

You may want to leave the church you are in, but never be a part of a church split. You will not prosper and every church that is born out of a church split will not prosper. It will split and re-split and split and re-split until the coming of the LORD, because there will be a spirit that rules in that church that is a curse.

If you want to leave a church, do it the right way. Do not burn bridges. Love that pastor, even if you do not agree with him for whatever reason, and communicate and let him send you out in *peace*. When you leave, do not be a *divisionmaker* and take others out with you. If a church is not ministering to you and your needs, find someplace where you can be fed, but do not murmur against that pastor.

Do not gather those to yourself
who agree with you
against God's anointed.

23) Immoderate Eating

Our bodies belong to the LORD, and we have a responsibility to give them proper rest, exercise and good nutrition. This is how we maintain our temples (our bodies) properly. We believe in good nutrition, and we believe in moderation (temperance).

> [19]What? know ye not that your body is the temple of the Holy Ghost *which is* in you, which ye have of God, and ye are not your own?
>
> [20]For ye are bought with a price: therefore glorify God in your body, and in your spirit, which are God's.   1 Corinthians 6:19-20

Our bodies are God's mobile homes. We must not take them for granted. If we will keep our spirits nourished with the Word of God and keep our lives free of devastating sin and occultism, and if we exercise wisdom in the care of our bodies, we will enjoy greater and greater measures of divine health.

Moderation is the key, in regard to exercise, rest or food. Moderation is one of the fruits of the Holy Spirit listed in Galatians 5:23 as "temperance."

If you are concerned about excessive weight gain, you should know, first of all, that it is a spiritual problem rooted in self-hatred. There is a spiritual root associated with weight gain.

24) Pure Unbelief

Because there was unbelief in the town of Nazareth, Jesus was unable to do great works in His own hometown.

> [4]But Jesus said unto them, A prophet is not without honour, but in his own country, and among his own kin, and in his own house.
>
> [5]And he could there do no mighty work, save that he laid his hands upon a few sick folk, and healed *them.*
>
> [6]And he marvelled because of their unbelief. And he went round about the villages, teaching.
>   Mark 6:4-6

There was unbelief in the Israelites coming out of Egypt. In Hebrews chapter 4, Paul addresses the issue of pure unbelief in those who came out of Egypt under the leadership of Moses.

Paul indicated that unbelief and doubt would keep us from our rest. Rather than believing and accepting what God has said, we try to create that rest by our own labors.

If fact, disease management is an example of man laboring to create rest by his own works. Disease management is a form of "works" that attempts to produce a rest apart from God.

25) Failing to Keep Our Life Filled Up With God

In John 5:14, after He had just healed someone, Jesus said, "Go your way, sin no more, lest a worse thing come upon you."

He was saying, "Keep yourself filled; do not sin." When God delivers you, you have an obligation to stay "filled up."

> [43]When the unclean spirit is gone out of a man, he walketh through dry places, seeking rest, and findeth none.
> [44]Then he saith, I will return into my house from whence I came out; and when he is come, he findeth *it* empty, swept, and garnished.
> [45]Then goeth he, and taketh with himself seven other spirits more wicked than himself, and they enter in and dwell there: and the last *state* of that man is worse than the first. Even so shall it be also unto this wicked generation.
> Matthew 12:43-45

It is important to note that when the enemy is removed, he will come back to see if you are "for real" and if you are "filled up" with the knowledge of God and obedience to Him. (See Luke 11:21-26.)

When the enemy is within you,
he is at peace,
and you are in torment.
Then when the enemy is gone out of you,
he is in torment,
and you are in peace.

26) Not Resisting the Enemy

In Isaiah 38:1-5 is the story of King Hezekiah who was sick unto death. The prophet told him he was going to die in his disease. He had a disease unto death.

What did Hezekiah do? Did he roll over against the wall and curse God? Did he roll over against the wall and go into abject bitterness? Did he roll over against the wall and have a pity party? Did he call the undertaker?

He prayed and he asked God for extended life. God heard him and healed him and gave him fifteen more years. If you have a disease unto death, talk to God! Ask Him for fifteen more years. You have a scripture to stand on!

One aspect of not resisting the enemy
is not asking God for healing.

The enemy is always trying to devour mankind through temptation, but the Scriptures indicate that you can defeat him and he will flee.

> [8]Be sober, be vigilant; because your adversary the devil, as a roaring lion, walketh about, seeking whom he may devour:
> [9]Whom resist stedfast in the faith, knowing that the same afflictions are accomplished in your brethren that are in the world.   1 Peter 5:8-9

> [7]Submit yourselves therefore to God. Resist the devil, and he will flee from you.
> [8]Draw nigh to God, and he will draw nigh to you. Cleanse *your* hands, ye sinners; and purify *your* hearts, ye double minded.   James 4:7-8

27) Just Giving Up

When you give up, you are believing everything the physical realm is telling you rather than pursuing healing. You resign yourself to illness when you focus on your symptoms, your prognosis and the word "incurable."

> [9]Mine eye mourneth by reason of affliction: Lord, I have called daily upon thee, I have stretched out my hands unto thee.
> [10]Wilt thou shew wonders to the dead? shall the dead arise and praise thee? Selah.
> Psalm 88:9-10

> What profit is there in my blood, when I go down to the pit? Shall the dust praise thee? shall it declare thy truth?   Psalm 30:9

233

Which is *a more excellent way* — premature death or a longer life in which to fulfill the will of God in your life? The LORD is more magnified in our healing than in a premature death.

> The days of our years *are* threescore years and ten; and if by reason of strength *they be* fourscore years, yet *is* their strength labour and sorrow; for it is soon cut off, and we fly away.
>
> Psalm 90:10

Remember, threescore and ten is seventy years. Did Moses say age 60 with some trouble? No! Did Moses say age 40 with some trouble? No!

He did not say age 30 with some trouble either. He says trouble does not start happening until age 80, then you have some trouble.

28) Looking for Repeated Healings Instead of Divine Health

Deuteronomy 28 says, that if we *disobey* the LORD our God, the curse comes upon us. If we *obey* the LORD our God, get all this stuff straightened out and keep working on it, He'll put none of the diseases of Egypt upon us.

Exodus says,

> And said, If thou wilt diligently hearken to the voice of the LORD thy God, and wilt do that which is right in his sight, and wilt give ear to his commandments, and keep all his statutes, I will put none of these diseases upon thee, which I have brought upon the Egyptians: for I *am* the LORD that healeth thee. Exodus 15:26

First Thessalonians says,

> And the very God of peace sanctify you wholly; and *I pray God* your whole spirit and soul and body be preserved blameless unto the coming of our Lord Jesus Christ.
>
> 1 Thessalonians 5:23

God's perfect will is not to heal you. His perfect will is that you do not get sick.

These principles will prevent diseases from ever coming in the first place if you will apply them to your life. Which is easier? Working this "stuff" out to get well or working this "stuff" out not to get sick? Both require fellowship, coming before God and being sanctified.

> Beloved, I wish above all things that thou mayest prosper and be in health, even as thy soul prospereth.　　　　　3 John 1:2

Is that His will for you? Yes, that is what it says in 3 John.

Do you think it is God's will to heal today? There it is in 3 John.

Do you think it is God's will that you be in good health today? It also says that in 3 John.

Do you think it is God's will for your poor head to be straightened out today? It is there in 3 John.

29) Rejecting Healing as Part of the Covenant for Today

In 1 Peter 2:24 it tells us,

> ...by His stripes we were healed.

In Isaiah 53:5 it says,

> ...by His stripes we are healed.

Psalm 103:3 says,

> Who forgiveth thee of all thy iniquities; who healeth thee of all thy diseases.

A lot of pastors today don't believe that healing is part of the atonement. They believe it passed away 2,000 years ago.

Wherever you are in your theology, whether you believe that healing is for today or not, if it's not for today in your theology, then it's not. Healing will never happen!

30) Trying to Bypass the Penalty of the Curse

Taking medication for a disease without taking responsibility for the sin issue behind it is trying to bypass the penalty of the curse. For example, if you have malabsorption because of anxiety, you have to deal with the root of fear and anxiety, which is sin. If you don't, then taking medication is an attempt to bypass the penalty of the curse.

The disease is the fruit of the sin. The fruit of the sin of fear and anxiety is malabsorption, and the drug is an attempt to manage it, apart from dealing with it. Another example is cancer, which results from bitterness.

We do everything under the sun trying to get well, instead of making peace with whomever we had bitterness toward. Making peace is dealing with the sin in the situation, dealing with the root cause.

Modalities of healing are an attempt
to bypass the penalty of the curse
by trying to get well
without doing it God's way
in obedience to Him.

This does not mean that people are never supposed to go to a doctor to find out what is wrong with them. What we are saying is that *if* your disease is spiritually rooted, healing or wholeness will come *when* you deal with the spiritual root through repentance and sanctification.

If you have this block, you are saying that you want your healing, but you do not want to go through the right doorway to get it. You do not want to go the route of repentance and sanctification. You would rather put your trust in doctors and medicine as an attempt to bypass responsibility before God for the disease, which is a curse in your life.

As the bird by wandering, as the swallow by flying, so the curse causeless shall not come.
Proverbs 26:2

Editor's note: Proper medical care, including diagnosis, is highly recommended. Doctors can safely maintain you while God is meeting you in your situation.

31) Murmuring and Complaining

Numbers 12:1-15 tells about Miriam's leprosy, which was a curse that came from murmuring and complaining.

Murmuring and complaining are signs of ungratefulness and will block God's movement in our lives. It can also open the door to bring destruction into our lives.

> ¹⁰Neither murmur ye, as some of them also murmured, and were destroyed of the destroyer.
> ¹¹Now all these things happened unto them for ensamples: and they are written for our admonition, upon whom the ends of the world are come. 1 Corinthians 10:10-11

> ¹⁴Do all things without murmurings and disputings:
> ¹⁵That ye may be blameless and harmless, the sons of God, without rebuke, in the midst of a crooked and perverse nation, among whom ye shine as lights in the world; Philippians 2:14-15

32) Hating and Not Obeying Instruction

The book of Proverbs says,

> ¹¹And thou mourn at the last, when thy flesh and thy body are consumed,
> ¹²And say, How have I hated instruction, and my heart despised reproof;
> ¹³And have not obeyed the voice of my teachers, nor inclined mine ear to them that instructed me!
> ¹⁴I was almost in all evil in the midst of the congregation and assembly. Proverbs 5:11-14

This teaching has come as instruction for you in righteousness, that you may experience *a more excellent way.*

Isaiah 28:8-19 establishes a plumb line for God's conviction to find its place in your heart. These verses sum up the entire problem of disease in the world and in the church today. page 312

33) Past and Continued Involvement with Occultism

Past and continued involvement in occultic practices, thinking or modalities of healing and disease prevention may prevent healing.

Occultism is mankind's attempt to heal himself and help himself. If we have followed these modalities we have opened ourselves up to occultic intrusion. We may have been following a mindset that is an abomination to God.

These philosophies, mindsets and activities are often an attempt to bypass the penalty of the curse without taking responsibility for the sin or spiritual defect that causes the disease.

It would be God's will
for you to be sanctified in these areas,
and not managed or manipulated
in your spirit, soul or body.

So teach us to number our days, that we may
apply our hearts unto wisdom.   Psalm 90:12

Our knowledge and wisdom come from teaching which is based on the Word of God, not the study of creation such as the sun, moon and stars. God has given us the hours, days, months and years of time so that in time (sometimes just in time) we may understand what He has said concerning our thoughts and actions, and not what a diviner, astrologer, soothsayer, false prophet or prophetess has said about the past, present and future.

Even in the church we have to have discernment in the application of the prophetic. Obedience is still better than sacrifice (1 Samuel 15:22), and sanctification and righteousness, including repentance from dead works (Hebrews 6:1), are still the foundation, not what the future holds.

When we exalt the wisdom of the "little g" gods, which are devils, insanity and mental confusion often come. When we seek the wisdom of this world, or the doctrine of devils, the Spirit of God departs. All that man has left is his own tormented mind, or a spirit of insanity from the devil. The first indication that the Spirit of God has gone is fear and torment (1 John 4:18).

The Bible gives us several examples where this happened:

King Nebuchadnezzar — See Daniel 5:17-21

King Saul — See I Samuel 28

Occultism offers to solve the problem. It always starts from a fear issue. Then it applies the enemy's thoughts and mechanisms to seemingly relieve the fear. But in fact, occultism offers no real solution, it only offers thoughts and actions that bring torment.

*The first line of defense against occultism
is knowing the Word of God.*

**Thou wilt keep him in perfect peace, whose
mind is stayed on thee: because he trusteth in
thee.** Isaiah 26:3

Many occultic modalities offer forms of spirituality, but lack the Word of God as a true foundation. They often use Scripture, but it is used out of context; or worse, used to manipulate or create future promises of blessing without any regard to righteousness, holiness and sanctification.

In conclusion, occultism always offers itself as the real thing from God when, in fact, the real thing is obscured and hidden. We are either establishing the kingdom of God in the earth, or we are establishing the kingdom of Satan through men.

Observable Characteristics
of Occult Bondage and Influence

Deep, deep confusion

Hatred of God

Distrust of God

Unable to sleep, night
torment, night terror

Hostility, aggression
and conflict

Fear of authority

Fear of relationships

Impatience

Control of others

Suspicion

Frustration

Insanity

Depression

Oppression

Tormenting thoughts

Certain types of pain,
especially in
relationship to the
central nervous
system

Feelings of isolation

Out-of-Body
experiences

Feelings of accusation
against others and
oneself

Divisionmakers and
troublemakers

Fear

Obsessions

Inability to hear God's
voice

Falling asleep in church

Falling asleep while
reading the Bible

Rebellion

Stubbornness

Disobedience to God's
Word...chronic
activities

Losing interest in
attending church
and reading God's
Word

Inability to develop a
prayer relationship
with God

Answers to Unit Nine

1. yes

2. yes

3. knowledge

4. knowledge

5. discern

6. forgive, forgive, forgive

7. knowledge

8. kingdom, righteousness

9. nigh, nigh

10. doubt

11. unbelief

12. hardened

13. hatred

14. tithes, offerings

15. fear

16. faith

17. troubled

18. hoped, not hoped

19. weak, sickly, sleep

20. believe

21. diseases

Study Unit Ten:
Closing Remarks

See *A More Excellent Way*™, 7th Edition, pages 317 – 322*

God will work in your life according to knowledge. What you have learned about roots of disease and blocks to healing gives you knowledge.

1.   Then, you can come before God according to knowledge and not according to _____.

Then The Holy Spirit can convict you and work with you, so that your life will be better. God is working in your midst according to knowledge, so that His good will may be performed.

In Nehemiah chapter 8:1-3 we get a picture of what happens when *conviction* comes.

> ¹And all the people gathered themselves together as one man into the street that was before the water gate; and they spake unto Ezra the scribe to bring the book of the law of Moses, which the LORD had commanded to Israel.
> ²And Ezra the priest brought the law before the congregation both of men and women, and all that could hear with understanding, upon the first day of the seventh month.
> ³And he read therein before the street that was before the water gate from the morning until midday, before the men and the women, and those that could understand; and the ears of all the people were attentive unto the book of the law.　　　Nehemiah 8:1-3

---

* Page numbers refer to *A More Excellent Way*™

The people gathered as one man (both male and female) and asked their priest to read the law to them.

2.   Were they in unity with each other?

yes ____ no_____

Ezra, the priest, read the law of Moses. Those that could understand were attentive.

3.   Could everyone understand?   yes ____ no_____

> ⁴And Ezra the scribe stood upon a pulpit of wood, which they had made for the purpose; and beside him stood Mattithiah, and Shema, and Anaiah, and Urijah, and Hilkiah, and Maaseiah, on his right hand; and on his left hand, Pedaiah, and Mishael, and Malchiah, and Hashum, and Hashbadana, Zechariah, and Meshullam.
> ⁵And Ezra opened the book in the sight of all the people; (for he was above all the people;) and when he opened it, all the people stood up:
> ⁶And Ezra blessed the LORD, the great God. And all the people answered, Amen, Amen, with lifting up their hands: and they bowed their heads, and worshipped the LORD with their faces to the ground.
> ⁷Also Jeshua, and Bani, and Sherebiah, Jamin, Akkub, Shabbethai, Hodijah, Maaseiah, Kelita, Azariah, Jozabad, Hanan, Pelaiah, and the Levites, caused the people to understand the law: and the people stood in their place.
> Nehemiah 8:4-7

4.   Did the people respond with sincerity and expectation?   yes ____ no_____

Their teachers, the Levites, taught them the meaning of the Word. Then they understood.

⁸So they read in the book in the law of God distinctly, and gave the sense, and caused them to understand the reading.

⁹And Nehemiah, which is the Tirshatha, and Ezra the priest the scribe, and the Levites that taught the people, said unto all the people, This day is holy unto the LORD your God; mourn not, nor weep. For all the people wept, when they heard the words of the law.

Nehemiah 8:8-9

5. Did the people begin to recognize their sins?

yes _____ no_____

²And the seed of Israel separated themselves from all strangers, and stood and <u>confessed their sins</u>, and the <u>iniquities of their fathers</u>.

³And they stood up in their place, and read in the book of the law of the LORD their God one fourth part of the day; and another fourth part they confessed, and worshipped the LORD their God.

Nehemiah 9:2-3

When conviction comes:

- We get the engrafted Word of God.

- We come before the LORD.

- We worship Him.

- Our hearts are circumcised.

Then we stand and take responsibility, not just for our sins, but also for the failures of our ancestors. Then genetically inherited diseases can be broken and the familiar spirits of our generations that rule us in our soul can also be defeated.

Editor's Note : See *A More Excellent Way*™, 7th Edition, Appendix C Walkout

Through A More Excellent Way™,
you have been given the Word
and the understanding.

If you want God to heal you
and deliver you from something
or to set something in motion
to bring change in your life,
take a little time now
and come before the LORD.

Confess the issues you are dealing with.
If you see these issues in your family tree,
bring that to the LORD and say,
"Forgive my fathers, also."

Refer to *A More Excellent Way*™, 7th Edition Ministry Prayer Model
in Appendix C, pages C-5 through C-7.

⁵And said unto them, Hear me, ye Levites, sanctify now yourselves, and sanctify the house of the LORD God of your fathers, and carry forth the filthiness out of the holy place.

⁶For our fathers have trespassed, and done that which was evil in the eyes of the LORD our God, and have forsaken him, and have turned away their faces from the habitation of the LORD, and turned their backs...

¹⁰Now it is in mine heart to make a covenant with the LORD God of Israel, that his fierce wrath may turn away from us...

¹⁵And they gathered their brethren, and sanctified themselves, and came, according to the commandment of the king, by the words of the LORD, to cleanse the house of the LORD...

³¹Then Hezekiah answered and said, Now ye have consecrated yourselves unto the LORD, come near and bring sacrifices and thank offerings into the house of the LORD...

2 Chronicles 29:5-6, 10, 15, 31

[25]...instructing those that oppose themselves; if God peradventure will give them repentance to the acknowledging of the truth ...

[26]...that they may recover themselves out of the snare of the devil...   2 Timothy 2:25-26

...let us cleanse ourselves from all filthiness of the flesh and spirit...   2 Corinthians 7:1

God does not require that we get sanctified all at once.

Then they killed the passover on the fourteenth day of the second month: and the priests and the Levites were ashamed, and sanctified themselves, and brought in the burnt offerings into the house of the LORD.
                2 Chronicles 30:15

Many of the people had not been cleansed.

[17]For there were many in the congregation that were not sanctified: therefore the Levites had the charge of the killing of the passovers for every one that was not clean, to sanctify them unto the LORD.

[18a]For a multitude of the people, even many of Ephraim, and Manasseh, Issachar, and Zebulun, had not cleansed themselves, yet did they eat the passover otherwise than it was written.   2 Chronicles 30:17-18a

Hezekiah prayed for those who were not cleansed.

[18b]But Hezekiah prayed for them, saying, The good LORD pardon every one

[19]That prepareth his heart to seek God, the LORD God of his fathers, though he be not cleansed according to the purification of the sanctuary.   2 Chronicles 30:18b-19

The Lord heard his prayer and healed them.

And the LORD hearkened to Hezekiah, and healed the people. 2 Chronicles 30:20

After this type of worship, the LORD *heard* the voice of Hezekiah and...

- He *honored* the voice of Hezekiah, and

- He *healed* the people

This is a powerful scripture of God's love, not only in the area of *total* sanctification, but also in the area of *partial* sanctification.

6. Did God pardon them and heal them even though they weren't completely clean? yes ___ no ___

Would you trust Him to do the same for you when you come before Him with a believing heart, expecting Him to meet you?

Pastor Henry asks God to meet you and to make the things that you are believing for your life begin to come to pass.

If you will do this, he believes that much of the oppression and depression and many of the things you are dealing with will start to change. He believes that because it is in God's Word.

Pastor Henry's Prayer

Father, I consider this a very sovereign time; I ask that You sanctify these people in the name of the Lord Jesus Christ, where they sit and as they come and where they're at...

I ask that You'll meet them in the integrity of their hearts and as they come before You, having heard the Word of God, mixing it with their faith, I ask that You hear them and receive their petitions unto You and forgive them their trespass and release them from the curse of their generations. I ask You this, Father, in the name of our precious Savior, our Lord Jesus Christ, as the work of the Holy Spirit. I release it, Amen.

Thank You, Father....

Lord, hear our hearts; hear our prayers...receive us. Hide not Thy face from us. Forgive us; release us from the sins of our fathers; forgive us of our sins and our trespasses as we forgive those who trespass against us. Lord, heal us; heal our families. Save us, oh God, save our families. We pray for our enemies and those who spitefully use us.

Lord, regard not the iniquities of Your people. May Your mercy and Your grace overshadow us. Heal us personally. Heal our marriages; heal our children. Heal our churches. Heal our political leaders. Heal our nation. God, let your salvation be spread to the islands of the sea from the rising of the sun to the setting of the sun. Let the earth be filled with the knowledge of the living God. God, we pray that this planet shall be inhabited in righteousness. Let Your Spirit move in our midst; convict us of sin; deliver us from all evil. Heal our land.

Father, I thank You tonight for being in our midst. Lord, be Lord of our hearts. We are Your people, the sheep of Your pature. Your mercy endureth forever. Blessed be the Name of the Lord. Thank You, Father... Hear our prayer, oh God. Send Your Spirit. Thank You, Father. We give You thanksgiving, Lord; we have not made ourselves, but You have made us. You are He that forgiveth us of all our iniquities and You are He that healeth us of all our diseases. You are He that daily loadeth us with benefits; yeah, even the *Elohiym* of our salvation. Lead us not into temptation, but deliver us from evil. Thank You, Father... In Jesus' Name... AMEN.